# WOMEN AND IDENTITY

# WOMEN AND IDENTITY
## Value Choices in a Changing World

C. Margaret Hall

*Department of Sociology*
*Georgetown University*
*Washington, D.C.*

●HEMISPHERE PUBLISHING CORPORATION
A member of the Taylor & Francis Group

New York     Washington     Philadelphia     London

**WOMEN AND IDENTITY: Value Choices in a Changing World**

1 2 3 4 5 6 7 8 9 0     B R B R     8 9 8 7 6 5 4 3 2 1 0 9

This book was set in Times Roman by Hemisphere Publishing Corporation.
The editors were Todd W. Baldwin, Mark A. Meschter, and Karla Philip. The typesetters were Linda Andros and Anahid Alvandian.
Cover design by Debra Eubanks Riffe.
Braun-Brumfield, Inc. was printer and binder.

**Library of Congress Cataloging-in-Publication Data**

Hall, C. Margaret (Constance Margaret)
    Women and identity: value choices in a changing world / C.
Margaret Hall.
        p. cm.
    Includes index.

    1. Women—United States—Psychology. 2. Identity (Psychology)
3. Social values. 4. Self-actualization (Psychology) I. Title.
HQ1206.H234 1989
305.42—dc20
ISBN 0-89116-785-4

89-7573
CIP

# Contents

# Preface

*Women and Identity* examines crises in women's lives as essential sources of personal growth and collective empowerment. Through its focus on women's historical subordination and the self-empowerment equality requires, it addresses issues related to the complex, sometimes incomprehensible human condition. A vision of women's potentialities and possibilities is proferred, with emphasis given to the initiation of the process by which women enter into full partnership with men.

*Women and Identity* is based on clinical sociological theory, integrated with life-history data from clinical and research settings. Because my purpose is to reach general readers as well as clinical specialists, an overview of these theoretical underpinnings has been placed in Appendix A rather than in the main commentary. I have worked as a clinical sociologist or family therapist in community mental health services and private practice since 1971. Ideal types—abstractions from the data—illustrate the most characteristic or dominant patterns of behavior in identity choices rather than specific case histories (see

Appendix B). Clinical data, interpreted against these ideal types, evince the variety of ways women pursue identity clarification and commitment renegotiation.

Clinical sociological theory applications generate significant explanations and predictions about women's empowerment processes and consequences. Although vision may frequently outweigh precision in this commentary, it is hoped that a balance has been struck in terms of the practical guidelines for women's everyday struggles. Taken together, clinical sociological theory, clinical data, and cross-cultural research show quite clearly the requirements and possibilities for women's private transformation and public empowerment.

Though values are difficult to measure and substantiate, an effort must be made because they permeate the dilemma women face. My hope is that *Women and Identity* will shed light on significant value choices for women, and contribute towards advancing the contemporary feminist enlightenment.

*C. Margaret Hall*

# Acknowledgments

There are many people to thank for their inspiration and support throughout the writing of *Women and Identity*, especially the women with whom I worked who described their lives so vividly. However, the main ideas for this book were consolidated during women faculty's efforts to start a women's studies minor at Georgetown University. I am particularly grateful to Leona Fisher and Sue Lanser for their interest in my work.

Less direct collegial exchanges sustained my writing. Other Georgetown faculty—Murray Bowen, Gwen Mikell, and sociologists in my department— listened and advised on the clarification of main themes for *Women and Identity*. Colleagues of the Sociological Practice Association also discussed my theoretical formulations, particularly Melvyn Fein and Louisa Howe.

Research assistants at Georgetown kept me up to date with feminist research and theory, and edited drafts of my manuscript. Kathryn Hughes, Katherine van Leuwen, and Rachelle Zowine all played important parts in shaping my themes.

Manuscript preparation was in the good hands of Samantha Hawkins, Kyong Pae, Janet Redley, Willy Hawkins, Veronica Cheney, and Maria Rezende. Their suggestions helped me to rewrite *Women and Identity* many times.

Publishing support from Bill Begell, Kate Roach, and Ron Wilder is much appreciated. These contacts link me to my reading audience, and their contributions make my work more meaningful.

Family members also inspire my work. My book could not have been written without the challenges of my husband, Robert Cole, and my mother, Madeline Hall. Much of my interest in saying something useful to the next generation comes from conversations with my daughters—Elizabeth, Tanya, and Jamy. Thank you all for adding much to my understanding.

*C. Margaret Hall*

# WOMEN AND IDENTITY

# Chapter 1

# Introduction

*Women and Identity: Value Choices in a Changing World* is based on the idea that we survive by aiming at our deepest, most meaningful fulfillment in daily living. Its primary objectives are to simplify and define patterns in complex facts, observations, and experiences, and to formulate principles and recommendations for action. We live in a world of ambiguities and must establish decision-making priorities that enhance the quality of life for individuals and populations.

The generalizations and propositions suggested here are based on clinical and research data collected from community mental health services and private practice in family therapy since 1971. The author has reported many of the findings from these longitudinal life-history studies at national family and religion research meetings.

Life histories are the primary source of information used. While specific cases are not included in the main commentary of this book, representative examples or ideal types are outlined in Appendix B. Emphasis is placed on behavior patterns that describe and explain shared experiences in identity empowerment and value choices.

The main generalization and assumption is that historically and culturally women have been socialized to fill subordinate and restricted roles. Stereotypes about women persist in most social settings as strong and even decisive influences in the values of both women and men. For example, a "good" woman is expected to conform to certain self-sacrificing, nonassertive, passive patterns of behavior. These models become standards that perpetuate women's subordinate roles. The highest status for women is still achieved through marriage. The roles of wife and mother are idealized and sanctified both in modern industrial and in less-developed societies.

*Women and Identity* addresses how women can challenge, neutralize, and modify the widely held social imperatives that restrict their mobility and fulfillment in society. A primary focus is how women can live more meaningfully through heightened identity awareness and more expansive commitments. Action flows from beliefs, and to the extent that women empower their convictions or "religions" about themselves, others ultimately become responsive and supportive of their new autonomy. Ways through which women can escape their confining roles are emphasized rather than the sources and nature of limited identity and entrapment.

There is much disagreement in assessing the gains of the feminist movement and in defining goals and strategies for advancing feminist interests. Drawing from clinical and research findings and historical trends, this book examines personal and social values in decisions at different life stages. The basic choices women make about work, marriage, and parenthood derive from their beliefs and values. Interaction is essentially negotiation or nonnegotiation with others' values.

We live in a world of assumptions and ideas. One significant determining influence in our lives is our understanding of human nature, from which flows our beliefs or "religions" about gender.

## SURVIVAL

Most women in the world live at levels of survival or subsistence. Their energies are consumed by making ends meet. Women have no time to call their own and little opportunity to assess the quality of their lives or status. Furthermore, they are socialized to accept restrictions and to consider themselves fortunate.

In modern industrialized countries, such as the United States, increasing numbers of women have sufficient time and energy for self-reflection. Even lower-class women in the United States have time and energy for themselves, although indigent women perforce are preoccupied totally with survival needs. When women have time to think and reflect about themselves and the world, they can develop a sense of who they are and cultivate this conscious identity. Women's education leads to fuller understanding, facilitating intellectual growth as well as social and cultural mobility. Education is one of the most significant means of women's entry into the public sphere. Learning about themselves and the world enables women to detach from the personal and private milieus of their family subcultures.

College educated women expect and demand more from life than did the previous generations of women in their own families. Education enables women to develop their potential and more accurately assess the requirements of a full life. By contrast, uneducated women are more likely to be forced by circumstances to wrestle with the grim necessities of their day-to-day existence. Educated women can afford to be less preoccupied with the mundane problems of making it through each day. As they become more aware of levels of human experience that go beyond survival, they generally seek increased fulfillment. If educated women aim only at survival, they deny themselves more satisfying ways of living. When women live only for survival, out of necessity they depend a great deal on others. Their neediness is felt keenly when relatives leave the family or die. When women know they cannot make it alone, they are obliged to ask others for help and sustenance.

Dependency has both beneficial and disastrous consequences. Women enhance their lives through the strength and support of others. They learn new ways to cope with harsh living conditions or effective ways to transcend their life situations. On the other hand, their dependency on others makes them increasingly vulnerable, and they may unwittingly subject themselves to others' abuse. Abused women may not survive these hazardous living conditions.

To the extent that the worldwide feminist movement has increased women's awareness of the abject living conditions of the vast majority of women, more privileged women realize that survival is frequently a monumental achievement. Although survival is necessary for a meaningful and satisfying life, this alone is not enough. To aim merely at survival is to expect too little from life. If women's life goals reach beyond narrow restrictions of current experience, their lives become more expansive. Being alive generates some tensions of striving, but women must gain a momentum that defines being alive as more than physical survival.

## FULFILLMENT

Fulfillment is an expansive awareness that calls forth our potential. It is the highest quality of life for individuals within a cooperative community. On a world scale, fulfillment is the cooperative community of nations.

When life is harsh and threatening, people who have goals beyond survival will be more effective and have more meaningful lives than those who are unable to see beyond the restrictive realities they experience. When we ourselves are fulfilled or strive for fulfillment, we become more able to assist those in need.

Women generally lead limited lives. Women of relatively high social status, celebrities, and professionals frequently lead restricted lives, as do those women more easily identified as unfulfilled. Women expand their horizons and develop their potential by making consistent moves towards fulfillment, rather than focusing on restrictions in extant conditions. Ideas and ideals serve rational or practical purposes for women's fulfillment. Ideals such as freedom lead to new opportunities and creative behavior.

Real progress for women is not merely opposition to patriarchal values of power and authority, although confrontation is sometimes a successful strategy for change. Women's challenge is to go beyond the status quo, to create structures and norms that do not merely adapt to existing conditions. By acting only in accordance with their own ideals, women transcend patriarchal values and develop cooperation and compassion. They are not fulfilled by modifying or destroying what exists around them.

Personal fulfillment implies contribution to the common good. We cannot realize our potential and live fully without considering and alleviating the suffering of others. Personal fulfillment requires that we examine our lives and reformulate our assumptions, especially where they circumscribe us. In order to create a firmer foundation for our lives, we must revise our understanding of human nature. Human nature need not be narrowly restricted. Cross-cultural research evidences the immense diversity in social conditions and human behavior. Although we have a few universal needs, and life moves towards fullness in a universalistic sense, specific human qualities and values show an infinite range of possibilities.

By moving towards fulfillment, women transcend empirical difficulties and survive. They survive as long as they aim for fulfillment. If they aim at survival, they perish in the long run. Many women are victims, and real shifts in their status can only be accomplished through cooperation with each other. They cannot lead healthy and meaningful lives in isolation from each other. They need other women to see themselves more clearly and develop strength and courage through their mutual support.

Whatever the restrictions in women's lives, one of the most effective ways out is to look up and forward to ideals they have chosen and with which they identify. Moving out of restricted existence occurs as momentum is increased by attention to ideals. Women must look beyond structures in their lives to accomplish effective change. Only when they live comfortably with their ideals can existing circumstances be transformed to the advantage of all.

## PATTERNS OF CHANGE

Searches for individual and social identity are unending learning processes that strengthen self. Identity empowerment is the successful outcome of search, research, and learning, whereby identity is clarified, deepened, and strengthened. Experienced by both individuals and groups, identity empowe_ condition of meaningful social mobility and improved social status.

Although each person's pattern of growth and identity empowerment is different, generalizations about regularities can be made. Sociologists construct theoretical or conceptual models called *ideal types* from these patterns. Ideal types are abstractions from data which represent the main characteristics of the phenomena examined.

One of the most distinctive trends in clinical and research data about women is that identity empowerment occurs when the primary domain of behavior shifts from domestic to both public and private milieus. As identity is clarified, women's traditionally circumscribed lives become dramatically less restricted. The frequency of women's interaction with others is exponentially increased through this empowerment process.

In patriarchal societies, women are restricted to subordinate positions in all areas of life. It is by making increasing numbers of deliberate value choices that women move into positions more equal to men. Women must move individually and cooperatively to their new territory of equality since men are reluctant to give ground with respect to their own superordinate position. The efforts of each woman are necessary to accomplish this kind of change. As no one person can make another person change, formal leadership in the women's movement is not necessary to bring about widespread shifts in status for many women. Women who strengthen their position cannot afford to ignore more dependent entrapped women. In order to guarantee their hard-won new advantages, they need to support and guide women who are not yet sufficiently free to act in their own interests.

Identity can be clarified most effectively through exchanges with others. Women learn a great deal about their own subordination and potential strengths by communicating their experiences to other women. Women discover their capabilities by listening to and identifying with women who cope successfully with social expectations and transcend restrictions imposed by themselves and others.

Another related pattern of change, which develops during the search and discovery of identity, is the emergence or deliberate construction of supportive contacts and networks. It is these kinds of structures that enable women to see themselves more compassionately through others' eyes, thereby understanding themselves and their motives more fully and with greater acceptance.

As women strengthen their identity, their roles become increasingly flexible. Instead of defining them in narrow, traditional ways, women begin to interpret more broadly roles, bonds with others, and expectations. Women no longer feel obligated, as did prior generations, to undertake responsibilities like child care. Traditional commitments are taken seriously, however, and new modes of behavior are developed to meet the changing needs and circumstances of families. This flexibility in role definition adds breathing space to women's stressful conditions of existence. Creativity is given to tasks previously accomplished in demanding and monotonous ways. This increase in spontaneity improves the quality of life of women and heightens their satisfaction. Such shifts in behavior move women beyond survival and towards fulfillment for all.

Although many more kinds of change can culminate in the identity empowerment process, the patterns described here represent the most basic changes. Tight sequences of events or segmented stages of development cannot be defined and conceptualized without losing some of the real-life aspects of experience. These models of change are primarily descriptive, implying explanation through references to value choices and negotiations of values.

## RELIGIONS

Systems of beliefs about gender differences may be thought of as religions. A deeper understanding of women and their subordination may occur from applying the concept of religion to particular values and expectations associated with each gender.

Values and beliefs about gender differences can be distributed on a continuum: traditional female values and beliefs at one end of the continuum and traditional male values and beliefs at the other. This mode of structuring diverse observations and assumptions about women and men demonstrates that complementarity and opposition occur between the two poles of typically female and typically male values. Tension exists between stereotypes or ideals of masculine and feminine values such as activity and passivity.

In the United States, many people's values fall somewhere between the extremes of female and male ideal types. In patriarchal societies female values are defined by men not women. When women in a patriarchal society gain status, they frequently espouse traditional male values as their own, though these values may be detrimental to their own interests: a ruthless female executive can treat her subordinates very harshly. Whether women accept and internalize traditional female values or traditional male values, they are vulnerable to the indoctrination of patriarchal values, frequently being victimized as a consequence of this dominance.

Values are central to life. We cling to familiar values tenaciously, and may cherish some values enough to die for them. As our innermost beliefs are the most intractable parts of our being, it is very difficult to change our values. We automatically internalize others' values in our childhood and youth. Adult maturity is the awareness of our own values, and their meaningful integration and incorporation in our lives. When we recognize contradictions and inconsistencies in our values and beliefs, we can modify or substitute our values by resocializing ourselves. Resocialization is an arduous, lengthy process involving extensive interaction with both supportive or nonsupportive others. Resocialization is akin to conversion, as we move from one set of values to another.

Our freedom rests in our ability to choose the values we designate as most sacred. To the extent that our values correlate with traditional religions, we will tend to be directly influenced by patriarchal values. When we define our identity and our gender autonomously, we detach ourselves from traditional patriarchal values and create new sets of values linking us to society in different ways. When the values we identify with form a coherent whole, providing us with answers to questions and concerns about ultimate reality, they can be thought of as a kind of religion. These new gender definitions and identities imbue our lives with moral power.

As women discover their most meaningful values and create real identities, they convert from ascribed religions of traditional patriarchal values about gender to achieved religions of egalitarian values. They move from the extremes of traditional female and traditional male values to a synthesis. Gender definitions shift into more general selections of values, and identity becomes androgynous and more autonomous. Traditional gender value systems are transformed by this process, enabling women to move from subordinated roles and restricted social positions to broadened opportunities for mobility and fulfillment. Women must honor and exercise the values of their new religions about gender by preventing former restrictive values from reappearing and exerting influence in their lives. This is accomplished by women's conscious cultivation of expansive values and by attention to the importance and significance of these values in their lives.

## NEGOTIATIONS OF VALUES

Our freedom is restricted if we allow our religions of gender or human nature to be closed belief systems. We must enter into extensive interactions with others to survive, to sustain a sense of self, and to lead a satisfying life. In these processes our values are negotiated with those of others, although our particular expectations and demands make other values nonnegotiable.

Women and men who are unaware of their values tend to accommodate other people, block communications, or withdraw from social interactions. These are reactions to the push and pull of values that they are not able to articulate or modify. A low level of awareness of one's values impedes the possibilities for equitable and meaningful relationships. When two people reach an impasse in value negotiations, there is a need to lower stress in the dyad. The tension is most effectively reduced by drawing a third party into this value negotiation. When negotiations between either member of the dyad and the third party work out, equilibrium in the three-member group is increased. If negotiations between each person in the original dyad and the new third party cannot be completed satisfactorily, another party is sought as a substitute third party to facilitate the value negotiations. When successful negotiations occur with the new third party, there is a reduction of conflict and tension in the dyad and triad.

Negotiations of values are basic social processes in small and large groups alike. Marriage and contractual agreements are long-term negotiations of values. Throughout value negotiations emotional equilibrium in power relations is sought on both conscious and unconscious levels, though there can be no definitive end stage of perpetual balance. In both micro- and macrostructures dyads tend to be unstable or "fluid," as one person can leave the relationship and terminate the dyad at any time. A triad is the smallest stable relationship system, enduring through consistent replacements of ineffective third parties.

Negotiations of values are the essence of social interaction. We express our primary values in meaningful interactions as well as ostensibly superficial exchanges. It is only when we deliberately choose the values with which we identify that our negotiations with others proceed according to our own interests. Women must have a keen sense of their innermost priorities in order to enter into negotiations that will enhance their lives. Intransigence in value negotiations is not evidence of strength or power. Although our values are nonnegotiable at particular times, a persistent unwillingness to compromise in relationships shows rigidity and intolerance. The repercussions of these attitudes and behaviors can be disastrously volatile or destructive. Maturity comes with the relinquishing of rigid, self-defeating attitudes and an unfeigned acceptance of the give and take of life.

Historically and culturally women have been both adaptive and submissive in their negotiations with men and older women. As mothers, women have usually transmitted patriarchal values through parenting, that is, in their negotiations of values with their children. It is only in recent decades in modern industrialized societies that women have refused to perpetuate patriarchal values, choosing instead to inculcate more androgynous and autonomous values. When women self-consciously select their values, they reflect their own interests more directly, thereby becoming stronger and more active participants in their future value negotiations. When women are more aware of what they really value, they are less likely to accept the dominance of patriarchal values.

Traditional cues and signals are no longer reliable guides to behavior in value negotiations between women and men. Women discontinue using patriarchal values as the central reference point of their lives. As women identify their own values more clearly and more consistently, they no longer allow themselves to be victimized by circumstances through series of ineffective, adaptive, and submissive value negotiations.

## FEMINIST GAINS

Feminism in the United States reemerged as a distinct social movement in the 1970s. In earlier periods, feminism was concerned less with values and the everyday behavior of average women than with specific goals such as legislative changes. Contemporary feminism in the United States and other modern industrial societies influences mainstream values, particularly those values related to equity. Although not unanimous in their goals and strategies, feminists work towards personal and social empowerment, cooperation and community. They promote alternatives to patriarchal systems of hierarchical difference, competition, and coercion.

As waves of feminism sweep through society, awareness within the general population is heightened. Women and men are forced to confront their differences, no longer finding it possible to deny or avoid issues. Feminism cannot be dismissed as an insignificant ideology that has little impact on people's lives. Feminism is a value and belief system that can be adhered to by women and men alike. Though feminism articulates the vital needs of any socially oppressed group, it is more likely to attract women as it attempts to address their real interests.

When feminism can relate to the basic needs of all women in all times and in all places, it will become a more effective social movement and will make considerably more gains. Feminism tends to be culture-bound and ethnocentric, unable to address the interests of the majority of women. Feminism has only begun to increase social awareness about equity and freedom. Gains achieved by feminism in the United States involve attitudes rather than behavior. Women are beginning to see themselves as equals. Acceptance of equality empowers women's identity, and this significant change in attitude is expressed in fruitful modifications of behavior.

Feminists have defined their grievances towards patriarchal dominance in compelling ways. When women recognize important nuances and complexities in the destructive conditions of their subordination, they are better prepared to survive and to overcome the personal and social consequences of patriarchy. Only when women define and confront their life situations can they establish realistic visions of improvements.

The feminist movement also has ameliorated suspicion among women and has eroded boundaries which historically cloistered women within kinship, ethnic, and socioeconomic groups. Women who are employed outside the home have to count on each other for support in domestic concerns and on the job. Prompted by economic necessity and intellectual interest, women cooperate with each other more than before, giving themselves added freedoms and options. Although there are still many gains to be made, some of the previous estrangements and perceived conflicts of interest among women have been reduced.

Women currently reap a variety of gains from the pioneering efforts of prior generations of feminists. Today's women do not need to create opportunities for advancement on all fronts. They can use their energies to contribute to continued progress rather than only make new beginnings. Though women may not be encouraged to develop careers by their families, the media and educational institutions communicate clearer messages of support than ever before.

Motivation is crucial for any realization of goals, and changing values increase women's motivation for personal and professional fulfillment. Gains need to be made in the relationship between women's personal and public domains. They cannot participate comfortably as equals in public life for part of the day and return home to domestic servitude each evening. This compartmentalization of roles and expectations persists in most women's lives, however, as they frequently assume full responsibilities both in the workplace and at home.

Fathers of daughters and men with spouses who work outside the home identify with some feminist ideals. More men are willing to parent actively today than in past generations, sometimes parenting daughters as enthusiastically as sons. Men may also be interested in and supportive of their spouses' careers, thereby furthering true community, friendship, and teamwork between women and men.

Feminist gains cannot be ignored or denied. It is a disservice both to women and men to overstate these gains, however, especially as they continue to be relatively small and modest. Much remains to be done in order to achieve a cooperative society with equal opportunities. It is in this broader, more ideal context that feminist gains need to be evaluated.

## GENERALIZATIONS AND PROPOSITIONS

Generalizations about changing values in the United States are suggested below. Empirical data outline particular trends and patterns in values.

1   The United States is characterized by different sets of values among varied social classes and ethnic groups.
2   Patriarchal values cut across all social classes and ethnic groups.
3   Patriarchal values derive largely from power phenomena and include most forms of authority, competition, coercion, and control.
4   Patriarchal values define and have a strong influence on traditional female values as well as traditional male values.
5   Secularization and modernization generate and give positive sanctions to alternative values to patriarchal values.
6   Equality is an ideological ideal in the United States, but there are large gaps between ideal and reality.
7   Value change at social and personal levels is slow, complex, and difficult to accomplish.

Propositions of ways to accomplish change follow.

1   Values are the most intractable characteristics of individual and social exchanges.
2   Patriarchal values have been automatically or unconsciously internalized.

**3** In order to cultivate values in their own interests, women must select values that expand rather than restrict their lives.

**4** By selecting values that are in their own interests, women strengthen their motivation and effectiveness.

**5** We are all equal participants in the human condition, and it is in everyone's interests to move towards autonomy and more general, less polarized gender definitions.

**6** Empowered women lead more satisfying lives and need to support other women and men in their efforts toward empowerment in order to be fulfilled.

**7** Survival can only be accomplished in the long range through fulfillment. We cannot live fully without aiming at ideals or moving toward our most satisfying goals.

# Chapter 2

# Women and Identity

Survival and the urge for self-fulfillment connect all of us at an irreducible level of humanity. Each of us reflects the collective, which in turn embraces the infinite diversity of its members.

As social beings our humanity is a product of interaction, not of isolation. The one and the whole are inextricably interrelated. It is when we discern this interconnection that we acknowledge our own duality as at once unique and universal. Individual identity is thus influenced by collective identity through the process of social conditioning. Identity arises as a product of our bonding with humanity. Equality underlies this unity of one and the whole. Each member is connected to the whole in the same ways as all other members—like snowflakes in a snowdrift or rays from the sun. We are equal participants in the human condition.

Interdependency is a central characteristic of human nature. Our interdependency defines our equality and our need for others. Interdependency is shared by all and it connects us at the deepest levels of self and emotional being. Our innate openness and vulnerability evidence this emotional relatedness. Emotional systems define and determine our patterns of interaction as well as our dependencies. Society and culture are built on human dependency.

Social environments are products of our negotiations and nonnegotiations of values, the components of our beliefs. When our values are negotiable we make compromises. When we refuse to negotiate our values we may continue to hold them to the point of death. These negotiations and nonnegotiations, or failed negotiations, create broader continuities and discontinuities in the values of our social environments.

Traditional and modern belief systems strongly influence individual and social behavior. For example, science has made many of us more materialistic. Beliefs and values are products of our social context, and each person is bonded to that context through their values and beliefs. Our cosmologies and world views establish patterns in our decision-making and life courses. A broader perspective on life allows us to see the details of our situations more objectively.

Individuals, groups, and society arrange values in hierarchies, some values being prized or cherished more than others. Shifts in these hierarchies of values create individual and social changes. Identity empowerment results from a realignment of one's innermost values, meanings, and contributions. This reordering of values must be conscious and deliberate in order to bring about long-term positive changes. Yet value choices are frequently not apparent to those who make them: we may automatically conform to or deviate from others' values. However, it is only through awareness and autonomy that we can self-consciously decide when and under what circumstances to conform or deviate.

Women have hierarchies of values that differ from those of men. Generally women value nurturing activities and sacrifice, whereas men value competition and dominance. Within the overall framework of women's values, varied ranges of values characterize different classes or ethnic and occupational groups of women. However, common denominator values, such as love, do cut across these subgroups of women, and are also held by men.

Identity results from choices. The clarity and effectiveness of our identity depends on whether or not we are aware of the choices we make. Identity is our closest personal link with social values. Due to the depth and intensity of interactive influences between self and values in identity processes, identity motivates behavior to accomplish ideals.

Women's identity has changed since the end of World War II: then family life and suburban living were valued, while today women value advanced education and occupational accomplishment. Throughout these changes, identity is a way to understand the being and activity of both women and men.

## CONNECTEDNESS

Human beings cannot exist in isolation from each other. People cannot be human without interacting with others. Life conditions include this necessity of being connected with groups and society. Our bonds with others are either life-enhancing or destructive. We enhance our lives and others' lives through our patterns of interaction with others, or we destroy ourselves and others through these exchanges. A common denominator of human existence is that we are bonded to each other. Connectedness between people is an essential aspect of our identity. Our shared heritage is that we are human beings rather than that we are women or men. Knowing ourselves includes awareness that we are equal participants in the human condition. Interdependency is a manifestation of this basic connectedness with others.

We cannot have a meaningful identity without acknowledging our emotional relatedness to others. Women need to know that they belong to each other, and that they have bonds with men. Women cannot be autonomous without realizing that they have a common destiny with all. Connectedness characterizes our layers and dimensions of self. Potential is developed through exchanges with others, and relationships allow us to lead meaningful and satisfying lives. We work towards goals and aspire to excellence through our social bonds.

We need a new way to think about our lives and the influence of society on us. We cannot understand human nature through concepts that suggest individuals are isolated from each other. Whether we like it or not, we must participate in diverse kinds of social organizations. We gain strength by deliberately constructing identities which acknowledge our connectedness with others.

One way to understand this connectedness is to view our relationships as systems. We are part of a whole, whatever its scope or range. A system can be a personal milieu like a family, a more impersonal context like a society, or the broadest frame of reference—evolution. A systems paradigm defines, describes, and explains characteristics of human relatedness. Understanding relatedness between women and men, and between women and women, is crucial for understanding all social systems in the human condition.

Feminists draw attention to the fact that patriarchal societies generate varying degrees of estrangement between women. In patriarchal societies most women are conditioned to attach themselves to men rather than to women, and these bonds to men generally restrict them. Women's distance and alienation from other women in patriarchal societies result from the central role men play in their lives. The resulting tensions generate conflict between women as well as estrangement, so they are unable to support and nurture each other.

In order to maintain a comfortable and rewarding position in a social system, participants must balance their autonomy and connectedness or dependency. Subordination between men and women expresses imbalance, and isolation between women perpetuates this imbalance. Men are understandably reluctant to give up what they believe are privileges deriving from their superordinate position in relation to women, therefore, they do not try to balance the social system. Women bring society's relationships into balance by breaking down their isolation from other women. When women identify their shared interests, they establish more viable relationships with each other. Women are empowered and supported through these relationships, and are able to change their patterns of dependency on men. Women become more equal to men by changing their relationships with other women. When women clarify identity and increase self-worth, they inevitably change their relationships with men.

## COLLECTIVITY

A collectivity is a group of individuals. Women and men are equal participants in the collective unity of life. Individual survival and fulfillment are inextricably related to the survival and fulfillment of the collectivity. Full being for women and men requires an awareness of their oneness with the human collectivity. The quality of our relatedness to the collective produces either fertile or sterile conditions for growth and development.

Theories of evolution and social change sometimes incorporate a principle of progress which implies an ongoing betterment of humankind in relation to moving forces. These theories tend to be so broad-ranging that they are frequently theological, philosophical, or ideological rather than accurate summations of reality. Scientific theories of evolution developed in Western social thought during the industrial revolution. They reflect cultural values of the West, such as unilinear or directional concepts of time, rather than the cyclical repetitions basic to Eastern thought. Whatever the broad view of society and individuals one chooses, varying degrees of connectedness between collectivities and their participants must be recognized. This connectedness precipitates regularities, patterns, and predictable trends in change processes.

Overall changes are difficult to observe, conceptualize, and understand. Evolutionary theories are becoming more accepted, gaining legitimacy as science. However, the human mind may never be able to grasp some of the predictable aspects of the broadest currents of social change. Applications of science to the study of human and social behavior are a relatively recent development, and the social sciences are still resisted by traditional disciplines and interest groups.

Given some necessary ignorance of evolution and change, we know that one characteristic of both women and men is interdependency. Collectivities form on a baseline of interdependency. Although mutual dependency is inescapable, we can improve the quality of our dependency on others. Autonomous bonding in collectivities is much more flexible and life-giving than the stranglehold of unquestioning conformity to stereotypes.

In all our transactions with others, we respond to the collectivity at some level of consciousness. We imagine we have an audience watching our daily activity, for example, although no one observes us directly. Dyadic exchanges are characterized by participants' awareness of others' expectations and social values. We aim for ideals and goals that reflect values of the collectivity rather than interpersonal needs. We aspire to professional success, rather than to completing one transaction with another person. We must honor the collective good, as well as support ourselves or sustain interest groups, if we are to be fulfilled. Complete action includes the collectivity and individuals. Women cannot achieve at the expense of others if their real interests are to be met. In large part current crises in social relations are due to the fact that men have tried to maintain and sustain their own goals, such as business profits, which are not directly related to the collective welfare. Men's behavior frequently negates human connectedness, dependency and needs of the collectivity, thereby undermining the social good.

By recognizing the importance of the collectivity, women build the kinds of communities necessary for social survival. Sharing child care and forming networks for professional development are examples of intentional communities. Freedom for individuals is increased through constructive and thoughtful interaction. Women change current patterns of human dependency in these ways, and larger numbers of people develop more fully. Nurturing activity is extended from family units to women's networks and communities.

## EQUALITY

The human condition is shared equally by women and men. Although it is difficult to specify universal characteristics of human nature, some basic needs for survival and fulfillment apply to all. We are creatures of habit and products of learning, and our conditioning must be both supportive and expansive. Social structures and social beliefs have created and maintained inequalities, such as those between different ages and ethnic groups. Although biological characteristics differ among individuals, these qualities in and of themselves do not make one group more or less worthy or more or less capable than others. Consciously and unconsciously we treat each other unequally in varied social contexts, especially when people in different classes interact. When emotional crises occur, we may address each other on more equal terms at deeper levels of connectedness. We experience these communications as more fundamental to our being than the social niceties and decorum of conventional everyday exchanges.

Although people may not be viewed as equal in aptitude, each has potential to develop, and a right to live as fully as possible. Equality may not be manifested in external appearances, yet the underlying reality of human relations is equality. We all participate in the human condition.

Historical records show inequalities in social conditions exist. A recurring pattern in most societies is the continued subordination of women to male power and authority. Women are treated as unequal in most social settings, and their activities are restricted to specific locales or functions such as childrearing. Women's narrow sphere of activity creates and perpetuates their isolation in society, generating imbalances in all social relationships. Society and individuals are harmed by these inequalities in being and in opportunities. One of today's pressing concerns is how to create the best living conditions for all people.

One major step towards realizing equality is to increase awareness about the inequalities that exist. Data show that in spite of legislative reform and increases in educational opportunities, many women are programmed and motivated primarily to fill subordinate roles even when their goals are of high societal value. Women's traditional values include respecting others before themselves; women do not exclude people from their idea of the common good; their conditioned thinking tends to be inclusive, considering all, rather than only themselves or an elite; and women also value cooperation as a means to achieve their goals, and as an end in itself. The increased empowerment of women will culminate in more assertion and a greater implementation of these values.

Women cannot depend on men to make changes in a direction of increased equality, especially when men do not view equality as essential to the common good. Men are reluctant to act in ways that appear to contradict their interests, and consequently resist increases in women's status. At this time in history only women can actualize the equality intrinsic to being human. People may deny or suppress equality, but each person has equal worth in spite of this denial. Women live equality for themselves, and serve as catalysts for others' realization of equality by holding their own in personal and public interactions with men.

## DEPENDENCY

Another approach to understanding the human connection is to define degrees of dependency. Dependency is felt, experienced, and enacted at different levels of need; interdependency expresses our equality of need at the deepest levels of being. Any quest for independence through identity clarification must acknowledge shared interests. These may include parenthood, education, or business. We cannot become more independent by isolating ourselves from others. In order to move away from socially imposed restrictions and develop our potential, we must see our needs in relation to those of others. Indeed, independence and autonomy are achieved only through action that accounts for our dependence.

Identification with collective values is a personal and social process directly relating to our connection with others. Increased awareness of our values enables us to trace the patterns of our dependency on others more clearly. When we see ourselves in this light—through the major trends of our connectedness with others—we may then ask ourselves whether we want to continue to live in these particular forms of dependency.

Patterns in our dependencies result from our own choices and decisions. Examination of the ways in which women identify with specific values demonstrates a wide range of choices and modes of dependency. We cannot choose to be totally independent from others, as dependency is an integral part of the human condition, but we can choose to increase or decrease the degrees and nature of our dependency. The negative binding effects of dependency are minimized by autonomy. In contrast, our most symbiotic, parasitical relationships with others culminate in extreme dependency.

Particularly strong dependence, such as intense togetherness with others, interferes with free action. This kind of dependency characterizes lower levels of functioning in the range of human behavior. Symbiotic, parasitical relationships are the least desirable patterns of mutual dependency, because they intensify limitations in behavior. Women's real interests must be promoted by achieving freer spheres of activity for themselves as well as their own goals. They cannot afford to invest all their energies in relationships with others.

Our identity is the source of the most significant ways in which we think and feel about ourselves. Identity is an influential psychic and social mechanism, and it motivates and guides our behavior. Personal identity is inextricably linked to social identity through the values we cherish. For example, we identify ourselves as Christian or Jewish in relation to social rather than individual beliefs. We do not consciously choose our original values, but rather automatically internalize those of others when we are young. However, in adulthood we can select different values to incorporate, or we can change the order of our preferred values. Value choices affect our patterns of dependency on others. When we deliberately change our values and priorities, our behavior and our inclinations to activity or passivity change. Behavioral problems and impediments in human functioning—for both women and men—can be traced to the values we draw upon for motivation. Values intensify the emotional tone of our relationships. Although our values tend to be intractable, objectivity enables us to choose them more freely. Increased objectivity enables women to become more autonomous, that is, interdependent rather than dependent.

## BELIEFS AND VALUES

Beliefs and values are products of the intellect and the emotions. Although beliefs and values may seem real to the individuals or groups who hold them, they are not part of an objective empirical reality. Researchers infer values from behavior, or analyze self-reports about values. Beliefs and values have essential subjective, inner meanings that cannot easily be observed, verified, or measured.

Our beliefs combine the facts of our lives in particular constellations, and select the facts to which we give our attention. If we believe families are important, for example, we notice events and characteristics about them. Our beliefs are both microscopic and macroscopic. We formulate our understanding of ourselves, of human nature, of life, and of the universe from the convictions which we hold most steadfastly.

Beliefs change during the different stages of our lives. However, some consider themselves adult in spite of their clinging to beliefs of their youth. Old beliefs become set and stagnant; closed beliefs rigidify and are perceived as facts. We may come to deal with religion as a thing rather than as a way of seeing ourselves and the world about us. Beliefs evolve from our values. If we perceive life as a process, for example, we will try to modify our beliefs and "grow" as the years go by. If we assess life as unchanging absolutes, we will not try to modify our beliefs and grow.

One consequence of our values and beliefs is that our relationships take on particular characteristics. Our assumptions about human nature may be based upon facts, but we come to believe people have certain qualities due to the influence of social definitions and respected values. Our perceptions of our- selves and others are frequently distorted. If we believe human nature is selfish, we see ourselves and others as selfish. We also justify the inequalities that we perpetuate by saying that this is the way everyone is. If we want to change our behavior, we must become more objective about our beliefs and values, espe- cially those about ourselves. We are influenced by the beliefs in our culture, and we tend to align ourselves with specific categories of social class, religion, or gender, but these statuses have behavioral expectations. For women, a common denominator of these expectations is that they limit and restrict their spheres of activity.

Changing our beliefs about life and how our environment influences us brings about changes in our behavior. We can choose to believe that we are actors in history whose lives make a difference, for example. Random, auto- matic, and erratic behavior is precipitated by restricting our lives through culti- vating passive or nonassertive values and beliefs. Changing beliefs is not an intellectual activity. This deep-seated process calls into focus and into question our most cherished values and definitions of reality. Our family relationships and social bonds are "cemented" by our beliefs and values, and our world views and cosmologies are sustained by them. The quality of our life experi- ence results from our beliefs and values. Our internal and external conflicts increase to the extent that our beliefs and values are inconsistent. Also, our values must be related to empirical reality in order for us to deal with others effectively.

We change our lives by reordering our beliefs and values, or by cultivating and strengthening new beliefs and values. Shifts in behavior occur when we bring our values into line with objective conditions in our lives. For women this process frequently culminates in their being able to take a leap forward due to increased faith in themselves. They are able to live more adventurously, with more risk-taking and more outreach to society. A revolution in the social order comes about through such inner and outer changes. Results are tempered only by immutable factors such as genetic heritage.

## CONFORMITY OR DEVIANCE

Choosing between values involves considering a continuum of possibilities ranging from conforming to existing values to deviating from existing values. The status quo is perpetuated by decisions to conform to established values and widely accepted patterns of behavior. A consequence of the decision not to conform is that new value systems emerge. This process of constructing alternative values and commitments is generally perceived and defined as deviance. When only a narrow range of conformity is tolerated by a group or by society, all wider ranges of behavior are viewed as deviance.

Women who decide to change or reorder their values, consequently moving away from traditional roles, are customarily perceived as deviant. Because this labeling is a negative sanction, it pressures them to move back to traditional patterns. However, in spite of continued widespread social expectations that women be confined to domestic roles, it is increasingly difficult for most women to conform to these restricted roles. As society changes, it is easier for them to deviate, and ultimately that deviance becomes conformity.

In some respects the choice to conform or deviate from traditional values is a false dichotomy. Most women both conform and deviate, frequently reacting haphazardly to the relentless sequence of everyday situations. However, this random decision-making is generally accompanied by conflicts and stresses. Society makes contradictory demands on women, such as expecting women to be frail and at the same time able to assume many grueling responsibilities. Women experience stress as they try to respond to these kinds of conflicting demands.

Women's heightened awareness of their values and identity allows them to become more autonomous in their decision-making. Their recognition of the conflict of values in their social milieus increases, and they identify more deliberately with values that have the most powerful personal and social meanings for them. There is much to be done to heighten women's awareness so that their freedom can be seized and realized in meaningful ways. Women cannot afford to cling to values which serve only purposes of the past. Orientation to the past, especially through commitments to stereotypical traditional values (such as being a good wife) produce much conflict and stress for women. When they try to honor only their commitments as a wife, they find that social structures no longer support this value.

Women need to acknowledge the influence of traditional values, but they must simultaneously resolve to move on and live their lives more fully than in the past. Women's private lives merge with their public lives. They are models for future generations, and their personal life-styles orient them toward possibilities for social contributions. Conformity to traditional values bestows some emotional security during periods of rapid change. Because women's moves to increased freedom are most effective and longer lasting when they are made easily and without impinging on others' lives, they sometimes choose to "go with the flow" of tradition to their advantage by consciously and deliberately deciding to conform.

Being perceived by others as deviant may indicate success in working towards more meaningful goals. Ideally broad social change includes basic shifts in traditions and norms, so women's "deviance" is gradually being accepted as responsible and appropriate behavior. Women have no control over public opinion, however, and it is essential that they persist in their pioneering attempts to modify or transform limiting aspects of their domestic responsibilities. They must be able to express their real interests by contributing directly to the collective good. Living fully necessarily includes community participation.

Decisions to conform or deviate are ultimately moral questions. These decisions have a powerful influence on women's physiology. Unless women learn how to assert themselves, they will manifest a variety of symptoms such as depression or cancer. If women fail to incorporate fulfilling goals in their lives, they will not survive in the long run. Their historical and traditional adaptations of fitting in or pleasing others no longer suffice.

## CHOICES

Women's options are extremely complex, being influenced by culture and class as well as gender. Summary points highlight a number of the dilemmas women face in their decision-making.

1  Traditionally women are taught to put others before themselves. However, in order to survive and be fulfilled women must center their lives on themselves rather than on others without limiting others' freedom.

2  Traditionally women have been pressured to put family living above other spheres of activity. Family living must be consciously and deliberately chosen rather than assumed to be the best option.

3  Marriage does not define all the life-chances of women. It is more important for women to come to terms with themselves than to search for the perfect or "right" spouse, or to consistently adapt to one's spouse.

4  Economic independence is important for all women and all men. Economic independence is conducive to emotional autonomy.

5  Life satisfaction moves in expansive rather than restrictive directions. If in doubt when considering strategies for action, move away from limitations and towards freedom and more expansiveness.

6  We are not defined by our roles. We exist apart from role expectations, and we cannot achieve goals effectively without stepping outside our roles.

7  Gender is learned. We can unlearn or undo inhibiting dimensions of our

socialization and programming by resocializing ourselves. Unlearning and re-learning make us more aware and stronger than if we did not examine ourselves and make these survival decisions.

**8**  Although we cannot decide precisely who we are, we can accept ourselves for who we are, and deliberately cultivate life-enhancing values or values we want to call our own.

**9**  Women need to resist automatically internalizing traditional male values as substitutes for traditional female values. Many traditional female values can be adapted to meet modern needs. Women must be themselves and in charge of their value choices at all times.

**10**  Choices are pervasive. Options can be discerned in any situation. No one decision is definitive. More expansive living means staying open to new options and choices.

Chapter 3

# Values as the Core of Identity

The quality of our lives is determined in large part by the values we self-consciously select and unconsciously internalize through our interaction with others. We consciously claim specific values as our own, incrementally defining and defending them throughout the course of our lives. In times of crisis we are asked to trade our lives and the lives of those we love to defend values seen by community leaders as decisive to the continued functioning of the collective.

Whether they be traditional or modern, our most important values may be internally inconsistent, reflecting the larger conflicts within an individual's society. Values are social creations existing well before and surviving long after individuals. Their perpetuation is ensured through the process of socialization, through which individuals internalize group values and the tensions surrounding them.

Families mediate the values of society. Parents consciously and unconsciously select the values they communicate to their children, who, because of their dependence, become participants in the parentally dominated family subculture. We come to know our values through painful experiences or behavior labeled by others as disobedient and nonconformist. We do not inherit gender-based social differences and expectations, but rather are socialized into them. In our earliest years we tend to absorb most of our parents' values. Girls learn how to be "good" wives, and boys learn that strength requires suppressing emotions.

Obedience and sacrifice for others are significant values in women's socialization. Such indoctrination makes it difficult for women to know who they are and to acknowledge their own feelings. However, women can resocialize themselves by changing their identity. Indeed, the real revolution is for women to transform their attitudes, behaviors, and the structures of society that restrict them. Women come into their own when they self-consciously accept or reject their parents' values.

Women need to consider both invisible and material realities. They can neither take from others to have their own, nor stand in the way of others. By virtue of their humanity, women are entitled to pursue their own interests. They are entitled to equal rights to live fully and to rewards for their efforts. As they become more alive, women become more autonomous. They need no longer merely conform or deviate, agree, or disagree. They carve out a niche for themselves in which and from which they celebrate life and inspire others. Women are empowered to serve those who need to be served, and are creative in all aspects of their lives.

Personal transformation includes sharing the means of fulfillment with those who desire fulfillment. Women multiply their life-chances by consciously identifying their own values, and they "come alive" by associating with those who already have the values they admire. In fact, meaning comes only through awareness, self-expression, and tolerance of others' values. Women cannot do this alone. They are only half of society and humanity. They must orchestrate their efforts with men so that they can cooperate rather than compete. Freedom starts within us, and women must use their freedom to free others, and become full members of the community of nations.

## VALUES

Values are defined in many ways and viewed from a variety of perspectives. Subjective components of values are embodied by individuals; objective components are manifested by particular groups or societies. We are strongly influenced by values, whether or not we are aware of such influences. When people make no conscious effort to choose their values, they internalize others' values and live in reaction to them. Awareness of one's internalized values is essential for meaningful living. Self is realized more fully by consciously and deliberately choosing values with which to identify.

When behavior is conscious and deliberate, values become ideals, goals, or principles. Some of our values are so deep-seated, however, that we may not be aware of their substance. For many of us it is difficult to acknowledge the strong influence our deepest values have on our behavior and on our daily expenditure of time and energy. Values are inferred from repeated patterns of behavior, interaction, and circumstances. Our values are clearly manifested by our interests. Values and valuating behavior tend to change through time. Maintaining flexibility in values has a distinct impact on behavior. Rigidly adhering to narrow interpretations of one's values at all times and in all circumstances results in restrictions, while flexibility in values leads to more expansiveness and satisfaction.

We tend to rank the importance of our values hierarchically. So long as the hierarchy of our values works well in our lives, there seems little reason to modify their order. However, when we cannot make sense of our lives, or when we experience pain in particular circumstances, we may begin to reflect on our values and possibly rearrange or change them. Crisis situations are particularly compelling, and they frequently reveal and urge new directions in our lives. Scrutiny of values and accurate assessment of their role are difficult to accomplish. We are not motivated to make deep-seated changes in our hierarchies of values unless we find no options for relieving discomfort. Crises, such as divorce or life-threatening conditions, shake the foundations of our being, necessitating radical adjustment or change. Personal transformation and social revolution result from reordering personal and social values. We identify with certain values, and our choices of values become our commitments. The quality of our lives depends on our values, and women's real transformation from imbalanced passivity to balanced activity happens when their traditional values are reordered, modified, or neutralized.

Social values do not generate balanced, harmonious relationships with each other. Value conflicts are common at both social and personal levels. Inner conflicts reflect or are generated by external value conflicts. We think our spouse always makes personal demands unless we realize the discrepancies between male and female values. When we nullify conflicts in our own value systems, however, we become more immune to value conflicts in the broader social context and more effective in our daily negotiations.

## BEING

Our awareness of ourself, others, and the world around us is an important part of our being. We experience anxiety when we allow others' values to impinge on our sense of self. In contrast, we find life satisfactory and enjoyable if we choose our own values and deliberately live in accordance with a set of harmonious values. Our most important values are ends in themselves, not means to ends. For example, we believe that it is important to love a child for no reason than that we choose to love. Happiness results from incorporating meaningful values in daily life. We experience well-being when we give attention to cultivating values we find significant.

Orientations and attitudes are other dimensions of being. The quality of our being determines our actions and accomplishments. We start from belief in a specific reality. Our actions are generated by this belief, and they in turn precipitate specific responses from others. Our social system is set in motion by our awareness of our innermost values and by our definitions of the nature of the universe. Others respond accordingly when we define situations as real. Restricted being generates self-centered activity, while expansive being inspires action that contributes to the collective good.

To a large extent it is a privilege to know ourselves. Self-cultivation has been historically viewed as the prerogative of those wealthy enough to keep at bay the mundane affairs of daily life. However, self-consciousness is not a luxury, but a common denominator of human survival which arises through adaptation to diverse environments. We observe our surroundings to assess them realistically and sustain our alertness, especially in circumstances that require us to modify our life conditions. Our being must be congruent with social definitions of reality in order to achieve effective adaptation. We cannot be so idiosyncratic in our belief systems that we isolate and estrange ourselves from others, but must be connected to live meaningfully.

One essential quality of being is open-mindedness to others. Our responses need to be flexible, and our relationships need breathing spaces in order to be truly viable, adaptive, and creative. Both women and men have denied the importance of women's being. Women may lose their sense of being through nurturing, caretaking, and supporting others. Only through becoming aware of the importance of being can women find and build identity. Knowing what they value is a way for women to get in touch with being. Times for reflection and contemplation are difficult for women to find in the course of their daily activities, but self-scrutiny is a necessity for living more deliberately and more fully. Being is not trivial or superficial. It is an essential component of coming into one's own.

## TRADITIONAL VALUES

Standards of behavior and ways to meet individual and social needs have been long accepted by people with status and authority. Specific traditions and values have existed throughout history. Social scientists have developed and refined the concept of role, distinguishing between traditional and modern expectations of behavior. Whereas modern roles are achieved, traditional roles are more often ascribed by conditions of birth. The underpinnings of consensus for women's traditional roles run deep, appearing in many different kinds of societies for long periods.

Women are strongly influenced by traditional value systems in all societies. Social values exhibit more conflict during urbanization and modern technological change, and women experience these as personal conflicts. For example, women's modern professional loyalties conflict with traditional family loyalties. Traditional values are based on the hierarchical ordering of authority and institutions in society. Some positions and functions have more status or power than others. The influence of elites in traditional value systems is legitimated by beliefs in "natural" inequalities, or by the widespread acceptance of authority structures that subordinate people. Traditional societies are characterized by repetitions of established patterns of behavior such as the succession of monarchs, or compliance and obedience to social imperatives. Attitudes here are unquestioning and conformity fairly uniform, that is, within a narrow range of accepted expectations.

Traditional values are difficult to change because they are focal references for established social meanings and explanations. Ongoing patterns of behavior are perpetuated by a belief that these patterns have always existed. The wellsprings of continuity, traditional values rivet women in their subordinate positions to men, although some women gain mobility by thinking and acting like men. Women in traditional value systems cannot have a full existence in their own right because their lives are not centered on themselves. They deny or ignore themselves in such societies, and are confined to caretaking functions as wives and mothers. Traditional values are passed from generation to generation as women transmit restrictive values to their daughters. However, most women are unaware of the extent of their participation in this generational repetition. They unwittingly limit their own lives and the lives of their offspring, and this behavior is reinforced by social processes and social structures.

Traditional values usually generate competition rather than cooperation. Frequently women do not have access to resources or rewards in traditional societies, except those related to their family roles and obligations. Thus, women are excluded from this competition. Traditional values demand unquestioning loyalty to patriarchal authority structures. Traditional value systems are relatively closed and resistant to internal or external pressures to change. They thrive best when the status quo is preserved for a long time, gender roles being clearly distinct from each other during these periods. Social institutions such as family, religion, and the economy reinforce traditional values and the subordinate position of women. In traditional societies they are either unpaid for their labor or restricted to low-paying jobs in the economy. Although there may be some breakthroughs in their social mobility, it is still quite difficult for women to change their roles in traditional societies.

## MODERN VALUES

Modern values emerge during industrialization and urbanization. Protestantism placed a new value on the individual, and the 18th century enlightenment emphasized the importance of freedom and reason. During the 19th century, people were no longer thought to be pawns at the mercy of historical forces, and efforts at social reconstruction in Europe raised hopes for democracy and intentional community. Science and modern values are historically related, as both developed during the industrial revolution when technology was used to raise standards of living. Scientific knowledge assumes universals in physical and social conditions. However, the accumulated data of world explorers and social scientists suggest much relativity in human values. Knowledge in the social sciences and humanities requires a broadening of definitions of human nature. In spite of these trends in discoveries, women were not a serious subject for systematic study until the 20th century.

Modern values became distinctive in a context of impersonal, densely populated urban centers. These conditions contrast starkly with the small community context of traditional values. Modern values include egalitarianism, but frequently this is manifested as ideal or ideology rather than as reality. The wide range of modern material values resulting from technological change intensified competition and motivation for upward mobility rather than increased equality. Achievement is increasingly possible and valued by large proportions of the population of modern societies. Roles and their limitations are no longer repeated through several generations, and both women and men have increased opportunities for career advancement and upward mobility, depending on their social class.

Pluralism characterizes modern societies rather than traditional societies, and wider ranges of cultural values are tolerated and accepted in modern value systems. Gender socialization is more fluid in modern societies, and male-female gender types less polarized. Gender differences may be acknowledged as learned rather than inherited. Authority and obedience are less valued in modern than traditional societies. In contrast, autonomy is valued more in modern value systems than in traditional societies. In modern times, patriarchal values are no longer accepted as fact, and may be both questioned and modified.

Modern values are secular rather than religious, secularization and modernization being correlated. Personal experience and individual feelings are valued in modern society, as is the quality of life at each stage of the life cycle. Family roles are strongly influenced by modern values. A typical middle-class family has two equal heads of family, or one single matriarchal head, rather than a patriarch who authoritatively binds all family members to his leadership and dominance. An important source of modern, increasingly secular values is the ever-broadening educational system. People are educated more as equals during the early years of formal education. However, college, graduate, and professional schools, although showing some increased gender and social class diversity in enrollments, reinforce gender and minority expectations prevalent in wider society by transmitting traditional values through their curricula. Goals of equality, frequently articulated as ideals of education, are slow to come into being.

Modern value systems are more flexible than traditional systems. This flexibility is in part created by needs to adapt to industrialization. However, due to ambiguities in expectations, flexibility in values frequently produces discomforting personal and social conditions. It is no longer clear what we should or should not do, although some of the same values are perpetuated in both traditional and modern societies. Our choices in values determine the quality of our connectedness with others and our behavior for personal and social fulfillment.

## VALUE CONFLICTS

As values diversify and multiply during modernization, newer values come into conflict with the more established values. Although wider ranges of values are tolerated in modern pluralistic societies, some values contradict each other or reflect incompatible differences. One value conflict in modern society results from a gender-based continuum ranging from typically feminine values to typically masculine values. Although women and men choose their own values more deliberately and more autonomously in current times than before, much socialization in gender roles and gender expectations is at unconscious or automatic levels of behavior. Women and men tend to react to each other in terms of gender stereotypes, especially when they have insufficient opportunity to reflect about particular situations or alternative choices. Another value conflict between women and men is the inherent tension between passivity and activity. Women have been programmed to be passive in most conditions, and men to be active. Passivity and activity are inadequate complements to each other as whole persons are the ideal. Furthermore, passivity and activity conflict with each other as directions or goals.

Historical and contemporary subordination of women result from women's and men's acceptance of the values of male supremacy and male authority. Authority structures in most societies are perpetuated by male leadership and female subordination, traditional male patriarchal values underpinning these structures. As modern values emerge, however, new and old values come into conflict, some conflicts being internalized by women and men as they deal with authority structures in their daily lives.

Belief in male supremacy is correlated with a variety of social and political advantages for men, and it is difficult for men to relinquish these prerogatives and strive for a more egalitarian society. Belief in male supremacy also has a negative influence on women's motivation. Women do not aspire to achieve social and political responsibilities traditionally associated with men because they cannot see themselves in these positions of power. One of the most basic value changes that could bring about major shifts in social organization is to increase the value women place upon themselves and upon the quality of their lives. It is not customary for women to place a value on their own priorities, goals, thoughts, ideas, feelings, plans, or aspirations. Historically and traditionally, they have sacrificed themselves for others, particularly for family members. Women frequently devote themselves to a lifetime of service without paying attention to their own needs or wants.

Women's habitual extension of themselves to meet others' needs has only recently been recognized as a dysfunction which may be both physiologically and socially problematic. When women cannot acknowledge the importance of self, their behavior becomes self-destructive, and directly or indirectly destructive to others—especially to their dependents. By not being actors women react to life, becoming victims of the push and pull of circumstances. Women meet others' needs and demands and ignore their responsibility for their own lives.

Clinical data suggest that value conflicts can only be resolved satisfactorily on a long-term basis when women increase the value they place on self, and select meaningful goals thoughtfully and deliberately. Whether women choose traditional or modern values, their decisions should be preceded by informed considerations of available options.

Value conflicts will continue in external social conditions, becoming more acute rather than merely perpetuating themselves at essentially hidden levels of reality. Women's challenge is to refuse to internalize society's value conflicts. Women need no longer be victims of circumstance. They can support sisters and brothers alike in acting decisively amidst social value conflicts.

## FEMINIST VALUES

Since World War II feminist values have emphasized women's experience and cosmologies. Feminist values characterize supportive, nurturing, life-enhancing and expansive dimensions of the human condition. The broad range of feminist values apply to all people—universal sisterhood, universal brotherhood, and universal humanity. They break through structural and hierarchical confines of patriarchal values. In contrast, patriarchal values reinforce authoritarian or stratified orders in social organization, these patterns being justified by history, tradition, and cultural context.

Feminist values imply a vision of universal community based on equal rights, worth, and opportunity. The most valued social process in community—cooperation—contrasts sharply with the competition valued in patriarchal societies. Feminist values emphasize pluralistic relations within the collective. Individuals and groups are perceived as being equal but different, and differences are respected, cherished, and lived comfortably and productively. Feminist values reflect the importance of being one's own person moving freely toward chosen goals. Freedom is a corollary of equality and social organization based on equal rights. Feminist values are expressed in political ideologies. They are distinctive values in that they link both private and public domains of activity. For feminists, the personal is political and the political is personal. People can no longer compartmentalize their lives in private-public dichotomies and survive the pressures of rapid change. What we tell our children in private must be lived in public. Women's contributions to society ultimately relieve the stresses and demands of their personal lives. They must integrate and consolidate personal and public values in order to retain a foothold on the moving sands of their day-to-day experience.

Feminist values are for the most part antithetical to traditional patriarchal values. Although the complexity of change processes cannot be explained satisfactorily, a feminist "tilt" of values in a direction opposite to patriarchal values is necessary before a more balanced, meaningful social equilibrium can be established. Recent shifts in patterns of family interaction in the United States, particularly since the 1950s, evidence the emergence of new values and related attempts to live more meaningfully. Although divorce and single parenthood have impoverished many women, there is an overall increase in opportunities for both women and men to live more freely. However, this hard-won freedom may not enhance the quality of life for most of the population. Also, on a world scale, most women do not yet recognize the disadvantages of their subordination to patriarchal values.

Feminist values must be applied to both small-scale and large-scale groups in order to achieve societal balance and fulfillment for the largest number of people. Small-scale applications may have to precede legislative change or other kinds of large-scale applications. When a sufficient number of individual women are empowered by feminist values, they will act on their vision of cooperation, and large-scale decision-making will become more balanced and enlightened.

One of the direct consequences and implications of feminist values is that barriers among women, among men, and between women and men, will be reduced or dissolved. New connections and more viable friendships will replace the isolation endemic to competitive patriarchal societies. Breaking through these frontiers realizes a society in which people can live together peacefully, meaningfully, and productively.

## GENERALIZATIONS AND PROPOSITIONS

A number of significant generalizations can be made about the central role of values in women's identity empowerment.

1 Values may be arranged along different continua. One example is to have life-enhancing feminine values at one extreme, and destructive masculine values on the other.
2 Values and valuating behavior are intractable aspects of human behavior.
3 Values are internalized consciously or unconsciously.
4 The influence of values on behavior depends on which values are inter-

nalized. While a value such as truth promotes questioning, values such as loyalty and obedience emphasize conformity.

5 We typically order values hierarchically, with our most significant values exercising the greatest influence on our behavior and decisions.

6 When values are reordered at individual and social levels, attitudes and behavior are transformed.

7 Identity empowerment arises from allegiance to particular values which give purpose and direction to daily activity.

The following propositions suggest ways in which plans for action can be based on the principle that values are the core of identity.

1 Values are social constructs agreed upon or desired by sufficient numbers of a population. We connect ourselves to others and to our goals through such values.

2 Our identification with values strongly influences our definitions of the universe and our assumptions about human nature.

3 Identification with specific values is a nonrational process that can be initiated by rational choice and self-conscious decision-making.

4 Awareness of personal and social values is a precondition of effective personal and social change.

5 Self-consciously choosing one's values is a powerful mechanism to precipitate personal and social change.

6 The substitution of life-enhancing values for destructive values results in identity empowerment.

7 If we choose to live fully, identification with life-enhancing values stimulates our efforts in this direction.

Chapter 4

# Changing Values in a World
# of Change

Values are the heart of human institutions. Social structures in various societies across time have been shaped by diverse value hierarchies. Individually and collectively, humanity selects values to live by and die for. Valuing is a necessary, vital process without which human life is incoherent. A so-called value-free existence is by definition antithetical to the human condition. Our degree of awareness and preferences notwithstanding, the substance and meaning of our personal and public lives are anchored in these social institutions. Values cannot be apprehended in neat and simple ways. We cannot meaningfully quantify value shifts even over the course of a single lifetime. The past and present diversity among public and private life-styles precludes a rigid definition of human nature and social dynamics. However, drawing from clinical studies and cultural research, it is possible to identify and compare individual and collective value patterns.

The quality of our lives depends on the values we hold and on our ability to express our values in everyday behavior. Secularization continues to move us away from traditional values and towards modern values. For example, patriarchal middle-class family values have been supplanted to a notable degree by more egalitarian expectations.

Value supplantation inevitably brings conflict at societal and psychic levels, as those with vested interest in the status quo resist the advance of less exclusive standards. The instability and moral whirlwind accompanying value shifts frequently results in the resurgence of traditional values. When social or personal crises threaten, we cling to the familiar for reassurance and meaning. When our values do not meet our intensified needs, however, we are compelled to reorder our values and priorities. Invariably, this process challenges our personal and social definitions of ourselves and the world. Thus, personal transformation becomes possible—perhaps even obligatory—through this process of value supplantation. The tenacity of social conditioning and depth of dependency cravings make such transformation a difficult and time-consuming process. However, we emerge from personal and societal crisis even more firmly grounded in spirituality if we do not resist instability, but rather negotiate it and allow it to modify us. Our resocialization is experienced as enlightenment, as it harnesses our intellectual, emotional and material resources for decisive action. Metamorphosis is achieved by resisting the pull of amorality on the one hand, and the beckoning warmth of inertia on the other. We reforge our relationships as a consequence of this metamorphosis. Awareness of our own values and of the interconnections of private and public, prompts us to extend the process beyond ourselves—first to our immediate circle, then to society itself. Indeed, we can create more humane, egalitarian social structures if we understand and accept our own and others' values.

## WORLD SYSTEMS

Changing values within society are understood more fully by considering the broader context of a world system. The term *world system* implies the interdependency of member nations, suggesting that societies shape and are shaped by their mutual interaction. Just as individuals thrive in a community environment, societies function in relation to each other. The interlocking components of the world system react to changes within the system by working towards a new equilibrium. Conceived in terms of this world system, value supplantation transcends economic, cultural, and religious boundaries.

Patriarchal values are pervasive throughout most of this world system. The institutionalized subordination of women to men is enormously resistant to change, given the commitment to the status quo of those who benefit from it. Throughout the world, only relatively small areas exhibit variations in this pattern of subordination. Furthermore, such variations as the rise of more egalitarian values are vulnerable to every political crosswind. The social advances accompanying modernization then tend to be claimed by traditional powerholders and dispensed piecemeal to pacify the "have nots" in their midst.

In most countries today, the expansion of world markets and the advance of industrialization have been accompanied by more egalitarian values. However, while homogenization of life-styles has diluted traditional mores throughout the world systems, in many instances distinctive and powerful traditional influences have been revived to cope with the political instability of economic materialism. In Middle Eastern societies, for example, long-established traditions have been revivified to buttress religious values in the midst of economic wealth. If no such concerted effort was made to uphold traditional, patriarchal values, they would be undermined by the egalitarian values and accompanying industrialization, and the materialism encouraged by enormous increases in national wealth. In many other societies, religion remains a powerful influence. Historically, religion is the original core of culture and source of traditional values. Religion legitimizes and perpetuates patriarchal values—the core of which is female subordination. However, secularization causes patriarchal values to lose much of their endorsement from religious institutions. Both secularization and modernization create significant shifts in the equilibrium of the world system.

While many societies continue to be rigidly stratified, with divisions resembling castes more than classes, contrasts have become less marked as universal education dilutes particularism and tradition. In spite of the opportunities offered by this increasing integration within the world system, however, women remain in subordinate roles. Class differences within societies separate women from each other, and even those women who have achieved professional mobility are accorded less acknowledgment than are men of lesser accomplishment.

## OBJECTIVITY

Objectivity is the impartial observation and sensory apprehension of the external world. Defined as a value, objectivity implies a broad understanding and a profound awareness of humanity's past and present accomplishments and travails as well as its future prospects. The prerequisite of value awareness and self-reflection is a capacity to step back from our ongoing emotional involvement with others and engagement in daily activity. Reflection about one's values and life course requires detachment and disengagement from routine.

Objectivity accrues through scientific knowledge as well as spiritual contemplation. This objectivity is necessary to understand women and their special concerns. Cumulative cross-cultural data place the lives of particular women across time and place into the context of world change. Objective understanding of women's subordination necessitates a reanalysis of completed research about women for contrasts among their experiences in diverse cultural settings. As well as facilitating a macro level understanding of women, this sort of objective base offers insights into micro level patterns of interaction.

In order to empower themselves through value supplantation, women must be sufficiently objective about their inner realities. They can only know their values through a detached appraisal of their acquired standards. Each must be assessed in terms of its substance and its advantageousness to further identity empowerment. Through identity empowerment, therefore, women come to terms with modernization processes, and with the nature of social change itself. Understanding social dynamics makes women more effective agents of change. They come to see the larger picture of their lives, to look at themselves as individuals and as vital members in a larger whole.

Objectivity can be cultivated and strengthened as a personal value as well as a personal skill. The more women can be objective about themselves, the more likely they are to be sufficiently free to move toward an equality which respects others. Objectivity helps them to be less reactive and it serves as a buffer to reduce stress in day-to-day interactions and demands. Objectively assessing their circumstances enables women to seek new options and opportunities.

## SOCIAL INSTITUTIONS

Social institutions are established ways for societies to meet their survival needs. Institutions are the core of all societies, underlying the vast range of different kinds of organizations within societies. Procreation needs are met by the family, and our needs to define reality are met by religion, although what constitutes family membership or how religion is defined is not universal. Knowledge is transmitted to future generations though educational systems, adaptation to the environment is accomplished through economic systems, and power relations are ordered through the political system.

The existence of social institutions suggests that there are universals in human behavior. The institutions of the family and religion are considered by some researchers to have existed in all societies at all times and in all places. Another property of social institutions is that they remain more or less intact throughout periods of social change. Without their effective functioning, societies are unable to exist. When societies become extinct, their demise has been attributed to the failure of one or two social institutions to meet basic social needs.

The values upon which social institutions are built are the most traditional values of a particular society. For the most part these values are patriarchal, perpetuating the subordination of women. Thus, it is at the level of the foundation of social institutions that values must shift in order for there to be widespread, accepted changes in relationships in society.

A society is a subsystem within the larger world system. Change in a social institution thus affects a whole society, and the world system itself. When family values in a particular society shift from traditional to modern, these changes have consequences for that society and for the whole of the world system. Although their lives are restricted, women are actors and participants in all social institutions in society. Though essential for the effective functioning of social institutions, women are subordinate or supportive to men in the roles they fill. The primary actors in social institutions are men. Women sustain men's activity by their passive assumption of private milieu nurturing or subsistence responsibilities.

A gender-based division of labor characterizes all social institutions, division of labor being the source of most roles. The close relationship between division of labor and roles is self-sustaining. Roles and expectations are structured to meet division of labor needs, and roles and expectations are perpetuated by continuities in these needs. In preliterate societies identical roles and expectations, especially gender roles and expectations, are repeated through many generations. Purpose in life in preliterate societies is defined as a replication of the life cycle of roles and work of prior generations. By contrast, modern industrial societies exhibit much more variation in life-course patterns among different generations. The young no longer automatically repeat the roles and expectations of the old, and gender specializations of tasks are not as polarized.

Social institutions function differently for diverse social classes. The upper and middle social classes are firmly bonded to social institutions in productive and advantageous ways. For example, upper and middle classes benefit from further education. Members of lower classes, however, tend to be in more marginal positions of social institutions, sometimes being the unwitting victims of conflicts within and between social institutions. Members of lower classes are also less mobile due to their comparative lack of access to opportunity structures such as colleges.

Social institutions resist change, and any change within and between them is gradual. However, institutional arrangements may be disrupted by intense or violent conflict. These dramatic shifts frequently last only for short periods. In the long run established institutional patterns reemerge, and social institutions reassume their equilibrium. Identity seems far removed from the forces of social institutions, especially when identity is seen as synonymous with personality. As identity awareness and its attendant commitments increase social action, institutions may be significantly modified by sufficient numbers of changes in identity. Identity also transforms individual and social vision, having a distinct impact on the values of social institutions.

## MEANING

It is much easier to lead a narrow existence or survive harsh conditions when one's life is filled with meaning. Meaning transcends empirical realities and gives purpose to the most difficult circumstances or crises. Historically many women resort to crafting meaning into their restricted lives. Thus, we are responsible for the meanings we attribute to our existence. In many respects this can be defined as a responsibility to choose, find, or create meaning in our lives. A meaningless life is experienced as an unfulfilled life.

In times of rapid social change, traditional symbols lose their meaning and new symbols or meanings emerge gradually as substitutes. Symbols are not essential to meaning. One can have a meaningful life without being aware of symbols and their role in communicating meaning. Symbols crystallize or consolidate meaning, and allow more people to attribute shared meanings to the specific natural or cultural objects they use as symbols. For example, when female beauty is symbolized as frailty, this debilitates rather than strengthens women.

Symbols are a means to an end, and not an end in themselves. Meaning itself may also be considered as a means to an end, in that it changes with circumstances. We live more fully and more enthusiastically when we have meaningful lives, but our search for meaning is not our highest goal. When we live life on its own terms, our end is not merely to grasp and yearn for meaning, but to live as fully as possible and to give to others. If our primary mission in life is to find meaning, we could be quite satisfied with limited lives. For example, the validity women attribute to subservience to men restricts their lives. Thus, unless the value women place on their passivity can be changed or transcended, traditional meanings will keep women in their subordinate roles in society and the world system.

Changing values in today's world have undermined a large number of traditional meanings. Modern Western values of autonomy have shattered rationales of gender-based labor divisions and expectations. It is by valuing themselves as autonomous individuals, and placing a value on the self as inner experience consistent with outer activity, that women move into more egalitarian modes of relating to each other and to men.

Modern industrial society places an increased number of demands on individuals, so that primary values are no longer predictably concerned with maintaining traditional authority structures within the family. Contemporary economic needs increase the value women place on work outside the home. However, the additional income they bring in tends to be used to increase opportunities and assets for family members. Still, advanced education defines new career possibilities for women, and employment possibilities are valued differently by women today than in past generations.

New norms are forged by the middle classes in the United States. Many women have more meaningful lives when they work outside the home. Women's mobility is increased by their valuing college and graduate education, and by their efforts to realize that professional achievement brings them rewards that surpass low-paying jobs or unpaid domestic work.

The fact that meanings can be chosen deliberately raises questions as to which meanings allow women to live more fully. Religion is an important source of meaning. Religious belief systems motivate women and provide goals, sometimes encouraging their articulation of more expansive world views. Motivation through religious meaning is generally more powerful than social status symbols or secular beliefs. Religious meaning directs or supports women to transcend the confines of their lives, facilitating action towards the accomplishment of ideals.

Meanings shift on a world scale and have not yet resettled into recognizable patterns. These changes cause considerable ambiguity in values, symbols, and roles. Although some traditional, established meanings remain relatively undisturbed by world trends, most traditional societies tend to be relatively isolated from modern world markets. Eventually, worldwide modernization will touch and possibly transform traditional meanings.

## PREDICTABILITY

The social sciences are not sufficiently developed to generate reliable theories predicting social change. Specific outcomes of circumstances or behavior remain difficult to foresee or explain. Continuities in patterns of social relations have been identified, described, and conceptualized to some extent, however. Tendencies or trends can be delineated, and possibilities or probabilities estimated. Clinical data in longitudinal research on women's changes are derived from interviews, self-reports, and observations. Wherever possible, facts gathered extend over a lifetime or several generations of family members. In the special case of women, identity, and values, some basic patterns in chains of events can be defined and tentatively explained.

Though ethnic or social class identities of women differ, their identities in general tend to be essentially narrow and restrictive. Identification with any traditional values limits women's lives, keeping their activity confined to arenas of family and subsistence work. Traditional values endorse subordinate and supportive roles for women. When women change their identity by aligning themselves with expansive values, such as freedom and activity, they emerge from their subordinate positions and make more direct contributions to the collective good. If women consistently identify with expansive values, their lives will predictably be enhanced and more satisfying. Improved conditions in society promote increased freedom for both women and men.

Clinical data show that women's identification with expansive values leads to improved physiological functioning as well as to more effective behavior in relation to self, family, and social groups. Self-assertion through identifying with expansive values such as action or expression, improves women's relationships and self-esteem. Their identification with transcendent values allows them to detach from the narrow and restrictive meanings which maintain the status quo. In turn, changes in identity affect all broader social systems.

The predictability of these outcomes in change processes depends on the degree to which women can consistently and persistently identify themselves with liberating values. Identification processes are emotional rather than intellectual, and include imitation and other nonrational processes such as faith and conviction. Our concept of self becomes more sacred through our deliberate cherishing or nurturing of specific values. In order for identity to have an impact on our commitments and social events, the self must be deliberately aligned with durable or transcendent life-enhancing values.

Changes in women's identity cannot readily or ethically be legislated or coerced. When changes in identity do occur, however, behavioral consequences are predictable, and women's contributions to the common good are increased. As individual women's needs are met, they increasingly orient their lives to social needs, particularly supporting and freeing other women for more active lives. Predictably, women support each other more when they claim expansive values for themselves. Women must depend on each other to increase their motivation for improving the quality of their lives and related social conditions. Although men may make genuine efforts to understand women's concerns and be supportive of women's efforts to achieve equality, they do not make the enhancement of women's status a primary goal. Ultimately, however, in order for men to be free, they too must neutralize the emotional bondage and negative conditioning of their lives. Both women and men must free their own genders from limitations if we are to have meaningful community.

## CRISES AND CONFLICT

In order for real change to occur, crises and conflict must be welcomed and used for constructive purposes. Many kinds of crises and conflict result from changes in identity, but these are potentially constructive transitions rather than destructive occurrences. If we fear or resist change, crises and conflict become destructive for ourselves and others.

When a woman changes self through deliberately identifying with life-enhancing values, the people who are emotionally closest to her will be disconcerted by that change, and will predictably pressure her to change back to her old self and former behavior. If the person emotionally closest to that woman, such as her husband, cannot successfully pressure her to return to her former behavior, a third party will predictably be drawn into the two-person relationship in order to stabilize the conflict. This third party may be a relative or friend, or a professional, such as a therapist or lawyer.

Crises are often experienced in personal rather than social terms. Public opinion implies that women are personally responsible for the origin of their ideas and feelings, and that their thoughts and feelings are unrelated to the social systems in which they participate. More accurately, we allow our thinking and feelings to be colored or defined by our social environments. Our responsibility lies in choosing which of these thoughts and feelings we want to cultivate.

Crises in our families, in our reference groups, and in society may be automatically internalized and experienced as our personal crises. Our challenge is to distinguish the thoughts and feelings of others from our own thoughts and feelings. In order to accomplish this, we must first realize and come to grips with the extent to which we are products of social programming. Having accomplished this, we can move into increased autonomy in our decision-making. If we examine our values in the context of larger social issues, we see that many crises and conflicts we thought were ours, which we allowed to define our personal lives, are in fact clashes or inconsistencies in society's values. Marital strife, for example, is frequently a product of incompatibilities in female and male socialization, or a result of tensions between demands of the workplace and family needs. When we understand crises and conflicts in this way, we articulate more viable possibilities for human relations.

The fact that women have historically and traditionally lived in confining conditions does not mean that subordination is intrinsic to society or human nature. Crises and conflicts can facilitate transitions to more egalitarian societies. Documented examples of women's transcendence of limitations and development of potential allow us to realize the latent power of women, and the ways in which crises and conflicts can bring about change. Crises and conflict are particular patterns of negotiations of values between individuals or groups. When values are nonnegotiable, crisis and conflict emerge from the impasses. Values are frequently nonnegotiable as they are nearly intractable aspects of human nature. In these respects many crises and conflicts are generated by a changing world.

Compromising one's values does not necessarily smooth negotiations, or even lead to fewer crises and less conflict. Compromise is essentially adaptive and passive behavior by the person or group who relinquishes values in the negotiations. Thus, unless life itself is honored by our open and free expression of values and commitments, giving up values ultimately intensifies crises and conflicts. Persistent compromise contributes to the volatility rather than flexibility of interpersonal relationships. Women have habitually compromised more in their negotiations of values with men than men with women. Compromise has historically been an integral part of women's adaptiveness and passivity in social relations. Women's challenge is to realize their lives more fully by expressing their values openly without allowing crises and conflicts to destroy them or others.

Potential for crisis and conflict is omnipresent, and we need to allow these to emerge if we are to grow. Crises and conflicts will manifest themselves as identity changes, and we must know and practice ways to deal with them constructively. Whatever the particular crises and conflicts in women's lives, they need the courage to continue to identify themselves with expansive values, simultaneously respecting and cherishing others for who they are, and their equal rights to life and self-expression. Active attitudes are not easy to acquire, but they create the substance of goals that take us beyond makeshift, piecemeal coping, and beyond perpetuating inequalities in the status quo.


## GENERALIZATIONS AND PROPOSITIONS

A number of significant generalizations can be made about the nature of changing values in a changing world. These descriptive statements give a broad picture of the complexities of social changes.

1  Values are a basic component and integrative aspect of societies and the world system. They are the substance of consensus, cooperation, and conflict in social systems.

2  Individuals and groups negotiate values with one another, forming patterns in social interaction.

3  In order to realize ourselves fully, resocialization is necessary, particularly when our values are restrictive and destructive.

4  Interpersonal and personal conflicts reflect and express value inconsistencies in the broader society.

5  Social change generates crises and conflicts in values which people internalize and experience as self-generated.

6  Worldwide change affects all societies in contact or communicating with each other. Over time, even relatively isolated societies are influenced by such worldwide changes.

7  Increases in the expansiveness of women's values increases the quality of their lives, and their values become more expansive with increases in their quality of life. Restrictive values promote only restrictive conditions, underachievement, and maladaptive behavior.

Propositions move closer to explanation and prediction than generalizations. A number of propositions suggesting relationships between various aspects of individual and social reality follow.

1  Identity is a personal and social mechanism through which individuals and groups promote and accomplish individual and social change.

2  Identification processes include a deliberate selection of values and alignment with these values. In times of rapid change, values multiply in number and diversity, becoming ever more difficult to define.

3  In times of rapid change, the importance of selecting one's own values increases. Unless women become more aware of value choices and make deliberate selections of values, their lives are subjected to the contradictions and conflicts of values in society.

4  Ideally, change produces new syntheses in society rather than new imbalance or a return to the status quo. Enlightened decision-making that promotes change is based on a vision of what a world could be rather than the historical facts of past societies.

**5**  Changing social values precipitate refusals to accept established modes or stereotypes of gender polarization. Women's freedom increases men's ability to discover their real interests. Men themselves need no longer be victims of power structures and materialism.

**6**  If we are to survive in the long-run and be fulfilled, our search for meaning in a changing world must be related to life-enhancing and transcendent values.

**7**  Change will subsume women's lives unless they become active partici- pants in the process. Through increased self-respect, women become agents of change rather than pawns of fate.

# Chapter 5

# Belonging

Each of us is an integral part of the universe. As members of society we inevitably have an impact on others—our lives have real consequences. We have deep-seated needs to express our belonging to society without limiting or harming ourselves. Fulfillment arises from our interaction with others for mutual survival and well-being. Our self-conscious membership in society facilitates these interactive processes.

Interdependency expresses itself in a variety of ways. We respond to others with symbiotic or parasitical behavior and automatic animal reactivity, or we pursue ideals and goals through objective reflection and independent behavior. Even when we are at our most autonomous, bonds with others direct or sustain us at deep levels of value consensus. Our socialization and environmental conditions define many aspects of our life situations. Being human necessitates that we consider and respond to standards and patterns in others' behavior.

We are most able to be ourselves with those we care about, although openness does not necessarily characterize our most intimate relationships. We establish our autonomy or dependence in the dyads and triads of our primary groups. Dyads are intrinsically unstable, as one person can end the relationship at any time. We form triads or three-person relationships to stabilize our dyads, especially when conditions of tension or stress exist in a dyad. Dyads and triads are units of our intimate relationships, and units of our modes of belonging to others.

Our strongest family relationships and friendships are flexible bonds—ties with breathing spaces. We benefit from intimacy where relatives and friends come and go in our lives. It is tightness or absence of meaningful ties in personal relationships that becomes problematic and imbalanced.

Distance in personal relationships is deceptive. In spite of an ostensible absence of instability, reactivity in "distant" dyads and triads is latent and can erupt unexpectedly through a large number of "trigger" events. Distance stresses relationships, making them volatile. The most advantageous conditions for belonging, then, are those which are flexible rather than reactive.

In order to understand the habitual ways in which women interact with others, it is useful to examine their patterns of interaction with members of several generations of a family. They can avoid the tendency to repeat these patterns of behavior by understanding their positions in these networks, and then by altering repetition by refusing to meet others' expectations. For example, women can break a trend of early marriage or early childbearing in a family by making different decisions than those of earlier generations. Women negotiate their values with others in new ways, and they reorder or change the values they transact with others.

Women need to feel that they belong. They must share aspirations to bring about equality, and build supportive networks. By selecting meaningful reference groups to enhance the quality of their lives, such as membership in political or professional groups, they restructure their activities and society in more effective and congenial ways.

Women's support systems develop their own subcultures and world views. Women's choice is whether to affiliate with long-standing, established traditional groups or to create new groups. Identity is forged through belonging to overt and tacit groups.

Women need support to modify their social functions. They speak more effectively for their real interests when they are organized and act collectively. Even when women manage to live autonomously, they must satisfy their deep-seated need to belong. They cannot live their lives in a vacuum, and choosing the nature of their dependence is a condition of their freedom and basis for increasing the expansiveness of their commitments. Thus, negotiating the tension between dependence and interdependence is crucial to women's individual and collective fulfillment.


## WOMEN AND BELONGING

To a great extent women belong to the same social class. Although empirical distinctions can be made between women in upper, middle, and lower socioeco-

nomic strata, the common denominator of their subordination is a significant
dimension of unity among them. This is true whether or not women acknowledge this unity. Men's interests do not allow women to experience the unity that
exists among them. Patriarchal values such as materialism isolate women from
one another and create mutual antagonisms among them. They are treated more
as objects than subjects and are seen as assets or liabilities that symbolize the
economic class or status of men.

Men cannot afford to support women's efforts to cultivate their unity because a breakdown in isolation among women jeopardizes men's hold over
them and men's superordinate position in society. Women's unity reinforces
their real interests, thus strengthening their social status. Unity among women
also leads to more satisfying lives on both personal and occupational levels.

Awareness of this commonality of experience and need is an essential aspect of being a woman and living fully. The metaphor "sister" is used by
feminist groups to connote this unity. Women belong to each other by virtue of
their similar physiological and social life conditions. Feelings of belonging
provide the support and strength necessary to women's survival and fulfillment.

Belonging ultimately means that the isolation women experience, however
powerfully perceived, will be recognized as illusory. In patriarchal societies
women experience psychic isolation from one another although they may work
in the same field or factory. Furthermore, there are very few settings where
women can meet to examine similarities in the limitations of their lives. Thus,
women's groups are needed to give support and direction to women.

Modern industrial societies provide increased opportunities for women to
heighten their awareness of the conditions of their mutual connections. Education, professional groups, and feminist exchanges allow more open discussion
about women's status. More women reach out to each other in supportive ways,
particularly within the middle class. Upper-class strongholds remain exclusive
and relatively impervious to these changes, while the energies of lower-class
women are dissipated by subsistence struggles.

It is significant for women to know, feel, and experience their unity across
time and distance. They cannot live fully when they are isolated from each
other. Furthermore, isolation strengthens men's domination over them. When
they are unable to communicate freely with each other, women cannot begin to
define and work for their interests.

Women belong to each other in the present, past, and future. Repetitions in
women's subordination to men can be traced throughout history, and only wom-
en's greater awareness in the present will modify these patterns for future generations. In order for women to make effective, long-range changes to enhance
the quality of their lives, they must understand their past and present circumstances. When they know their historical roles and expectations, they realize
how deeply entrenched restrictive values are in their conditioning. No major
changes can be made in these powerful processes until women understand more

about who they are and who they have been. Awareness of a shared heritage can bring women together to increase their strength.

Belonging and needing each other are not signs of weakness. On the contrary, it is when women do not recognize their interconnections with one another that they weaken themselves. Acknowledgment of their affinities moves them towards individual and collective identity empowerment. Belonging provides support and strength for more expansive commitments.

## IDENTITY AND BELONGING

Identity is a mechanism which balances individuality and togetherness. Though denoting individual characteristics, identity combines personal uniqueness with social qualities. Our identity derives from deeply held values and beliefs about ourselves. Self-concepts and related behavior are defined emotionally rather than intellectually.

Women's knowledge of their own distinctness and difference from men strengthens the unity among women. In this respect identity becomes an essential aspect of women's effective belonging. For women, identity is a source of both strength and weakness. If women believe that they exist only or largely to serve men, every aspect of their lives is colored by this. As a source of identity, then, this belief makes women willing and eager participants in strengthening patriarchal values in society. In contrast, if women believe that they exist in their own right and have a responsibility to live fully, their identity and behavior are transformed accordingly. Identity defined by this belief encourages women to work to supplant patriarchal values with more egalitarian social standards.

Belonging frees women when their identity is clarified and consciously shared with other women. The substance of women's identity—their uniqueness and distinctiveness—vitalizes their unity or belonging to each other. Identity differentiates women from men and enhances rather than limits women's lives. Paradoxically, women are both like and unlike men.

Identity results from the value choices women make throughout their lives. Awareness of their unity affords women more options, as they identify and emulate the professional and personal transformations other women have accomplished. As members of the human race, both women and men can choose expansive opportunities and expression.

People have contradictory needs—the urge towards autonomy and the craving for symbiosis. Identity synthesizes these diverse tensions in our lives. We identify the self as unique, and at the same time identify with other people or groups. We are in charge of our lives when we both act independently and deal effectively with others.

Women need to distinguish the ways in which they identify constructively or destructively with others. If they choose to identify only with traditional patterns and influences, they may cultivate a sense of belonging to class. Upper-class women's lives are frequently restricted and half-li... small proportions of women appear to have many material advantages, but there is a higher price to pay for their limited roles and conditional approval. Furthermore, their material advantages are frequently bought at the expense of the well-being of lower-class women. The quality of life of those who work to support the life-style and daily activities of upper-class women is reduced by the monotony of their tasks and low pay.

Identity gives most meaning and efficacy to unity when it defines women and men as equal participants in the human condition. Women and men belong together as humans. They cannot afford to fight or destroy each other, as they cannot impair each other's freedom and at the same time live meaningfully and with satisfaction.

Identity concerns suggest that women must be selective and deliberate in the ways in which they define their mutual connections. However, they should not shortchange themselves by sharing with women without a particular strengthening purpose. It is women's responsibility to themselves, and to future generations of both women and men, to acknowledge their links with other women in order to achieve vital and expansive goals. Women reinforce each other through their interaction and interdependency. Identity and belonging are thus mechanisms that foster mutual awareness and simultaneously promote re-assessment of conformity to traditional expectations.

## BELONGING AND VALUES

Belonging implies consensus or agreement on shared standards and values. We need each other for empathy and support at both physiological and emotional levels of being. The ways in which we see ourselves and others in relation to these needs are the substance of our values.

Our reactivity and emotional dependence can be channeled by a conscious, deliberate cultivation of values that transcend our survival instincts. Our membership in humanity is aligned with our self-image and the esteem we afford others; that is, understanding our equal participation in the human condition brings with it an awareness of the importance of respecting others, whether or not they share the same beliefs and standards.

If interdependence is viewed simply as the survival of a particular society, shared social values will be parochial rather than universal. Adherence to narrow ranges of culture-specific values, such as particular status indicators, leads to conflict. A broad range of values is essential for creating and sustaining a sense of belonging to humanity and to the universe.

When we change our values, then, we change the scope of our interrelations. The different groups to which we belong or aspire to belong are reference groups—groups that we value, are emotionally significant to us, and form foundations for our identities. When women choose to move beyond restrictive roles, their reference groups—college, graduate school, or professional associations—become broader in scope, and their sense of belonging moves from domestic areas to historical or universal contexts.

Our belonging in these broadest contexts is described in many ways. Universal values, such as love, are defined in their particulars to the extent that they enjoy cultural diversity. Only when such widely shared values are flexible and tolerant can they continue to have universal applications. Narrow and rigid values—such as sectarian religious dogma—tend to be subsumed by more inclusive and expansive values.

Women's lives are strongly influenced by the values of their immediate milieus. Their belonging to each other in a universal context must also be expressed through the values they choose in shaping their identity. Although the vast complexities of change processes essentially lie outside the control of women, each woman can empower her identity. Women help each other to broaden their interdependency and strengthen their effectiveness. Ultimately, these shifts have a direct impact on society. When women enlarge their vision and the scope of their behavior, they broaden their interrelationships and create models for other women to emulate. They may choose not to imitate each other, but their reasoned deliberation and consideration of options necessarily acknowledges the increased possibilities that exist due to the efforts of other women.

Values generate patterns of behavior. Women modify the ranges of their behavior when their commitment to specific ranges of values changes. New patterns of activity emerge as women change their habits of thinking about themselves as someone's mother, daughter, or wife. Women are human beings with essentially the same rights and privileges as men. Each life has consequences for others, and it is our responsibility not to impinge on the lives of those with whom we interact.

Identification with idiosyncratic values generates isolation and conflict or combativeness. Identity is more effective when values reach beyond the singularity of the individual, creating a breadth in understanding and communication. We negotiate values with others more satisfactorily when we share the same or similar values. If our values set us apart from others, negotiations become difficult or impossible.

Outreach and value sharing are structures of empowerment. Alienation, powerlessness, and meaninglessness characterize isolated living. Idiosyncratic values do not integrate with others' values. Established values—such as knowledge—make interaction more effective and more meaningful. Widely accepted values facilitate exchanges and negotiations because there are more shared interests to transact. Broad bases of values empower people who share the same values because security, recognition, and self-esteem are the results of mutually satisfying negotiations.

Sharing values becomes problematic when identity has no conscious distinctiveness; people need both to conform and to deviate from norms. We establish our own meanings in the context of meanings we share with others, but we need to hold certain distinctive values as our own.

Women belong to each other in the world, not merely in specific social settings. Narrow ranges of values are not functional for women when they participate in settings beyond domestic milieus. Narrow standards restrict women's lives and must be replaced by more flexible universal values to erode limitations. Values of tolerance and respect give creative breathing space to both women and men, and they facilitate the modification of existing standards and expectations.

## BELONGING AND CHANGE

Our bases of belonging are at the core of our personal and social identities. Belonging provides a foothold for women during times of rapid social change. They accomplish personal changes more effectively when they have a clear sense of belonging. Our bases of belonging are at the core of our personal and social identities.

Belonging derives from a group's consensus of values. Each member's values must conform with group values to some extent in order to define membership in that group. As our values change, our membership changes from one group to another, or from one position or status within a group to another. We seek to perpetuate our security in social relations by seeking membership in substitute groups. Personal changes generate shifts in group memberships.

Societal changes disrupt established value systems, the foundations of many reference groups in society. As individuals are affected by changes in both societal and smaller group values, they lose their sense of connection. These shifts are disconcerting, but the resulting increase in fluidity and flexibility provides an opportunity for the establishment of new values.

The increased population density in our industrialized and urbanized areas creates impersonal social conditions. Mass society and bureaucracies have replaced communities. It is easier to become isolated from others when we do not know the people with whom we interact. Part of the challenge of adaptation in modern society is to find meaning amidst the impersonal norms of city living. In spite of dehumanized social conditions, it is possible to bring purpose and direction to daily activity through identity expressions. Only when women deliberately chose their values and pay consistent attention to identity concerns can they neutralize anonymity and cultivate purpose or direction in modernization processes. Women can be overwhelmed by others' demands and by their inclinations to conform to others' values and standards. Constant compromise and adaptation to external demands enfeeble women. Thus they empower themselves and attain satisfaction or dignity only when they exercise choice in their values and identity.

Women's roles and expectations have been remarkably resistant to social change. From a broad historical perspective it is only very recently that women have begun to question their role in society, or make changes in their behavior. Attitudes have impeded change, and approval of women's subordination has maintained these inequalities throughout industrialization and modernization. Resistance to examining values and identity has also produced resistance to change. By contrast, exercising choices in values and identity initiates change. Once new views of life and life's responsibilities are formulated, behavior shifts beyond established roles, ultimately having an impact on the whole of society.

More equal participation by women and men increases societal equilibrium. Technological society is in danger of destruction or extinction, and women's more peaceful, nurturing values can emphasize new social priorities. The infusion of women's qualitatively distinct values in existing patriarchal systems promotes new syntheses and structures, while the status quo perpetuates existing restrictions in women's lives.

Belonging for women is a powerful aspect of change. If women continue their allegiance to traditional values, remaining loyal only to their families, expansive social change will be precluded. When women formulate newer, freer values and expand the number and scope of their reference groups, their role in social change will be more active and constructive. Women can invite the kind of change they prefer by shifting their group memberships to contexts which are more supportive of their fulfillment.

Women's belonging to each other does not exclude a consideration of men. Women must emphasize their own needs and aspirations, however, in order to deal with the entrenched patriarchal values that surround and permeate their lives. In contrast to masculine values, such as competition and material acquisitions, feminine values generally include concern for men.

Change occurs whether we desire it or not. Women only realize themselves fully by taking an active role in cultivating those changes that are in their interest. Belonging gives women power and creates more possibilities for using power.

## HARMONY AND CONFLICT

As women carve out more advantageous niches for themselves, they increase their mobility in society. Their moves follow triadic patterns in interaction and negotiations of values since triads are the most stable units of their new networks. When women are upwardly mobile, they generally change their group memberships along traditional lines. Though they seek to meet the different standards and expectations of a higher class, they continue to conform to tradi-

ince women's individual needs are generally not met by established val-
/hen modes of belonging deviate from established traditions, short-run
uences are conflict-ridden and long-run consequences are potentially har-
us and in the interests of all. Our choice is to know and decide the price
ll pay for social harmony.

armony and conflict are not fixed stages or end points. Harmony and
t reflect possibilities of social arrangements as people negotiate values
ach other. When negotiations of values break down, relationships move
nflict or estrangement. Compromise or agreement in negotiations culmi-
in social harmonies. Belonging is an integral part of the sequence of
that culminates in harmony or conflict. Conflict may result from har-
however, just as harmony may result from conflict.

## LEVELS OF BEING

ging is a social mechanism that allows us to change our being or aware-
s we deliberately exercise choices in our identification with others. If
n affiliate with nontraditional groups, they reach new levels of being. If
n affiliate with traditional groups, they perpetuate their subordinate posi-
nd expectations.

ew levels of being bring satisfaction and fulfillment, but they cannot be
ed without shifts in values and social structures. Deliberate attempts to
identity are necessarily accompanied by corresponding changes in group
ions. Our modes of belonging, such as reentering the labor force, expe-
d reinforce new levels of being.

embership in increased numbers of interest groups characterizes new
of being for women. Their awareness widens to include social class
ership and participation in history. Restrictive beliefs are examined and
ulated, particularly those that are reinforced by established religions.
imes this scrutiny motivates changes in group affiliations. New self-
s and world views actively influence our lives. This more profound un-
nding motivates decisions to diversify or substitute memberships in
s, thus neutralizing restrictions in women's lives.

ansitions to expansiveness in identity are accompanied by new, more
tic goals and structural shifts, such as social mobility. Belonging is a
ness that balances this tendency towards mobility. We all need roots and
ctions in our lives, and we benefit most from cultivating connections with
s which allow us to move and thrive.

ur interdependencies must be flexible. We need togetherness and autonomy
l growth and development and the fruition of opportunities in our lives. In
to stay socially mobile, we must be able to change memberships in our
nce groups. We may need to be able to shift our positions between central

tional values such as low ambitions and self-sacri
harmony in our daily lives, excessive conformity is
sonal fulfillment. Traditional values restrict both wo
their social contributions. Decisions producing harm
tably produce disharmony in the long run if they res

When women decide to experiment by incorpora
lives, they extend their activity from neighborhoods
New loyalties and affiliations produce new strains ar
are divided between home and society. However, a:
longing are chosen deliberately, not blindly, the nev
more integrated with women's real interests and exp

Belonging to nontraditional groups, such as ne
autonomous values and standards for women which
procedures. Changes in women's behavior are resist
tionally closest to the women making changes, and
those relationships then become manifest.

This interpersonal conflict may be short-lived. V
new modes of belonging eventually sustain their pe
comfortably or break away from them. Separation ar
these breakdowns. Women who resume some tradit
frequently do so in new ways. Interpersonal harmony
women cannot compromise themselves—this merely
flict resulting from new modes of belonging subsides
if women persist in their newfound autonomy. Shoi
structive; these disharmonies open up new possibilit
Shared expectations change, and spouses are given m
to explore possibilities for relating and living. Conflic
bility for ossified, rigid customs. This allows interest
New modes of belonging, such as women supporting
phase in this chain of events, as is identity empoweri

Harmony and conflict are consequences of shifts
of individual women and their collectivities. When
organization, such as a professional or political grou
derstanding of themselves, their society, the world, a
en's collective views and visions run counter to tradit
ion and the legal or political establishment pressure
former subordinate status. Ultimately, women as a
accepted and harmoniously integrated into society. Cl
would require the supplantation of traditional restrict
by more flexible and egalitarian beliefs.

Modes of belonging generate either harmony or
which conform to established values has immediate h
for society. Such adaptation tends to give rise to confl

ever,
ues.
conse
monic
we w

H
confli
with
into c
nates
event:
mony

**NEW**

Belon
ness
wome
wome
tions

N
achie
define
affilia
dite a

N
mode:
memb
refor
Some
image
dersta
grou

ideali
roote
conne
grou

for fu
order
refer

and marginal locations in the groups to which we belong. This change in status in relation to our groups increases our autonomy and functioning effectiveness.

New levels of being result from membership and loyalties in imagined groups as well as visible groups. We do not need formal association or membership as much as identification and imagined connections with others who are alive or dead. We must feel that our rootedness and connections are real, but it is not essential that the group with which we identify actually exists. Imagined groups and ideals need to have some basis in reality, however, such as a group from the past, or a group which is unapproachable. Invisible groups that are remote from reality, such as populations from another planet, become isolated fantasies rather than bases for new modes of interaction.

Women's self-consciously chosen identities produce new levels of being. Chosen values create new structures in women's lives, such as different familial and occupational roles. New individual patterns of behavior are integral parts of broad social change processes. Being actors rather than reactors makes women's behavior qualitatively different. Placing a value on truth and knowledge rather than on tradition, for example, opens up possibilities for innovative change.

Our interdependence is such that we cannot get beyond our needs for group membership and group interaction. Maturity includes choosing groups that support our long-range interests and goals. Our belonging and interaction with these group members solidifies our connections with others, and we function more effectively in our daily lives. More expansive levels of being enhance the quality of our lives. New being generates visions of individual and social fulfillment, and these ideals function as meaningful goals. Expansive being increases possibilities and advantages for all women and men.

## CHOICES

We need groups in order to be fully human. Isolation is ultimately destructive to self and others. In modern impersonal social conditions, it is frequently necessary for people to make conscious and deliberate efforts to cultivate their awareness of belonging to groups in order to create meaning. Freedom includes deliberate choices in belonging to groups which enhance and multiply our opportunities. Freedom and reason are vital for women's escape from entrapment in narrow roles.

Our options for establishing interdependencies and connections include the following.

1   We choose to belong to groups that promote our expression and growth, rather than groups that restrict our thinking and activities.

2   We choose to become more aware of the groups to which we already

pay allegiance. Though it is not easy to know where our loyalties lie, we must scrutinize our preferences and our investments of time and energy.

**3** We choose to relate to groups autonomously rather than in overly dependent ways.

**4** We choose to persist in spite of the conflicts and pressures which predictably surface when we decide to belong to new groups.

**5** We choose to work for harmony in the long run rather than harmony in the short run, even though the former may be accompanied by a painful transition accompanied by conflict.

**6** We choose groups through the values with which we identify. Our values guide us to the groups which have the most meaning for us.

**7** Identity is strengthened by negotiations of values with others. Different groups engender different patterns of interaction. Triadic exchanges are the most stable units of interaction.

**8** Changing group membership is a means of social mobility. Upward mobility weakens identity when there is increased conformity to others' standards and values.

**9** Belonging may be associated with visible or invisible reference groups. Groups prominent in the past, or groups in distant places, may be equally or more influential and meaningful than groups in close proximity.

**10** Flexible belonging allows us to move between central and marginal group positions. We choose these positions depending upon our desire to conform or deviate from group norms.

Chapter 6

# Change and Evolution

As difficult as it is to describe social change, it is even more so to formulate a broader evolutionary perspective. Though the most significant forces in change may be discerned as patterns, they can be neither definitively proven nor predicted. Each of us needs to find our bearings and define reality amidst the flux of circumstances and interaction. We make assumptions about the nature of change and ourselves in relation to change. Once we have firmly grounded ourselves, we act according to our assumptions about reality, though we may be unaware of the influence our presuppositions have on our lives.

It is not as imperative for us to formulate assumptions about evolution as it is to have some understanding of social change. The immediacy of the latter gives it priority in our lives. By contrast, evolutionary processes are experienced as being so removed from our everyday decision-making that we generally assess human nature without using an evolutionary reference point. However, if we choose to understand evolution more fully, our understanding of ourselves will be enhanced. Evolution can be defined as specific values and qualities of being, as well as physical processes. We stabilize and orient ourselves in change and evolution by our deliberate and nondeliberate acts of identifying with values.

In order to live constructively, we must make decisions and commitments to invest our time and energy creatively. Our identities are forged through our daily interactions, and by our defining and moving towards specific goals. The groups we belong to, or want to belong to, give a sense of connectedness, community, and wholeness to our lives. It is through social integration that we become most functional. Individual and shared interests are realized more fully when women feel kinship with each other. Through the assistance of others we reinforce our individuality and achieve more. Thus, fulfillment derives from action which affirms values and meaning in everyday existence.

When we view our existence in relation to the cosmos, we get a clearer sense of our position and purpose in life. We are able to see ourselves as integral parts or dimensions of broad evolutionary processes at physical, emotional, and intellectual levels. We are also able to see our potential to participate in evolution more deliberately and more fully. From this broader perspective we discern an increased number of avenues of opportunity and mobility.

We change our behavior more effectively when we alter our perceptions of the personal and public milieus of our lives. Self-conscious redefinitions of our familial roles enable us to see the possibilities and limitations of our daily lives. Redefinition of our realities prompts us either to embrace more socially mobile patterns of behavior, or become even more comfortably entrenched in traditional modes and expectations.

In this process of cognitive and emotional change, women experience tension between their own and others' definitions of reality. They confront the fact that the innumerable acts that go into defining and responding to "reality" are individual and social enterprises. They realize that we construct our realities consciously and unconsciously, reinforcing or refining our values and perceptions in this process. For example, our understanding and applications of love is modified by others' reactions and responses.

It is our need to share cultural values that ultimately provides a source or basis for meaning, identity, commitment and rational action. Our capacity to be free and to reason evolve through individual and social expressions of the values we share with others. To live fully is to live more deliberately and more selectively. Purpose in life becomes more comprehensible and more attainable when we direct ourselves towards ideals rather than survival needs. Women can no longer afford to focus simply on coping or getting by. Putting all their energies into survival greatly limits their fulfillment. Furthermore, women will most certainly not flourish in a changing world unless they make significant progress towards their fulfillment.

## SCOPE

The issue of women and identity is not a narrow concern, but rather encompasses all aspects of change and evolution. Identity is related to the grand scheme of things—we can only fully understand ourselves when we apply these broadest possible perspectives.

The concept of social change can be applied to human societies more directly than can evolutionary theory. Whereas evolutionary theory attempts to describe and explain all life in the universe from a scientific viewpoint, social change is more readily associated with historical and intercultural comparisons. Knowledge of social change is a primary concern for women since cross-cultural research findings substantiate that women's subordination has been experienced by most women in most societies at most times. Consistencies in this pattern motivate women to pursue ways to modify those existing inequalities.

Theories of human evolution are not yet fully accepted as fact, but our species is changing gradually, developing new modes of communications. The human brain has increased in size and complexity during successive geological time periods, and future evolutionary trends may create new levels of human consciousness.

Studies of evolution do not generally include research about values except to document society's increasing emphasis on them in the later stages of human evolution. Social change research, by contrast, highlights the importance of values, especially the documentation of influences related to the rise and fall of civilizations. It is only in relatively recent times, however, that humans have moved sufficiently beyond immediate subsistence needs to be able to reflect on their lives with a degree of detachment. Knowledge and education broaden and deepen our understanding of the human condition and ways in which we value certain activities.

When our lives are repetitions of ascribed roles—imitations of the lives of our foremothers and forefathers—we necessarily have a limited awareness of the world about us, and no working knowledge of societal change or evolution. We are unable to define alternatives to traditional roles under these circumstances. When we are caught up in impersonal, compartmentalized living in modern urban conditions, we easily become estranged from our human heritage and from broader change processes. We appreciate and understand ourselves more fully only when we see and know the scope of life outside our own relatively narrow concerns.

Whatever the realities of evolution and change, our ideas about evolution and change have a decisive influence on our behavior. We can think broadly about evolution and the nature of human nature, while at the same time close our minds to the possibility of real change. For example, evolutionary theory may be narrowly deterministic, facts being interpreted as illustrating the instinct of survival of the fittest in and among societies. Other evolutionary theorists have more open definitions of change and formulate hypotheses based on human choice and the refinement of human nature through environmental influences and learning.

Social change theories have frequently been based on conceptualizations of societal repercussions accompanying the industrial revolution. Women and men are conceptualized not as the animal creatures of evolutionary theorists, but as materialistic beings who believe that progress is possible. Evolution and industrialization suggest different views of women. These are important in understanding women, even if that understanding is limited and more related to stereotypes than reality.

Physiology is emphasized in scientific theories of evolution. Explanations of industrialization generally incorporate emphases on materialism. Both of these major perspectives tend to exclude the full consideration of other formative influences on women and men. Women are more than biological beings with specific functions to perform, and more than subjects or objects of production and consumption. Our knowledge of change and evolution must include more comprehensive interpretations of the human condition. This knowledge of evolution and social change enables women to see the promise and limits of change more clearly. We cannot make changes outside the realm of possibility, but neither need we be confined by historical or evolutionary precedent.

## CONTEXT

Evolution and change are important aspects of a thorough examination of women and identity. The breadth of evolution provides a context for deepening our understanding of women. We put ourselves in perspective and gain objectivity by seeing ourselves in the broader picture of creation.

We cannot construct identity by assessing priorities in a vacuum. Identity cannot be an effective change mechanism when it is removed from reality. Our reality is shaped not only by immediate structures in our daily existence, but also by broader currents in life forces. Private and public milieus and environmental or evolutionary influences affect our being and behavior.

We cannot understand problems when we concentrate on them too closely. We must detach from them to put them into perspective. Fresh and effective solutions to problems are formulated when we enlarge our vision and put facts in this broader perspective.

Our values provide us with a frame of reference for understanding the world. Meaning derives from context. In order for women to select or create goals, they must see their lives in both an individual and social context. Although evolution and change may not be considered important by most women, if they can consider their lives in relation to evolution and change, possibilities for their fulfillment are enhanced. Options for women increase when the context of their lives is broadened. Vision is expanded when life situations are defined in terms of currents of change. For example, women decide to work towards a change in legislation when they see the broader picture of subordination.

An alternative context, less directly related to evolutionary change, is the course of a single life. We can translate our understanding of broad change processes meaningfully when we apply them to the whole of our lives. We see how the politics of specific decades change our thinking and point of view.

Effective decision-making and clear choices flow from a positive, strong identity. We can understand ourselves more fully by considering the nature of human nature through our knowledge of evolution or change. This also allows us to see our lives as products of consistent and deliberate modifications in identity.

Since we have no direct control over broad change processes, our scope for responsible action, and the most meaningful context for our decisions, is our lives. We establish our identity by making decisions about the whole of our lives. Our selection of values and identity is influenced by the context we use to make our assessments of the world about us.

Historically, women have made others central in their decision-making to the exclusion of themselves. They need to reexamine their decision-making processes and make themselves a primary concern in order to reestablish balance in interaction. They cannot allow the demands and expectations of others to move them from their solid foundation of self and identity in decision-making. If women put others into their context of decision-making, they must view them as equals, and as recipients of their action. They need to sustain equality and activity in their definitions of situations. Their decision-making will be more responsible when they keep their attention focused on what they can do in given circumstances, rather than allow others to define situations for them. It is their definitions of reality, and not others' definitions, that establish effective structures and contexts for their decision-making.

Neither all of the facts of a given situation, nor the exact nature of evolution and change processes can be known. Given these limitations, human beings symbolize their understanding of these broader realities. Symbol systems include science, religion, art, politics, literature, conventional social class cultures, ethnic groups, and gender. Symbols open up immediate empirical dimensions of our lives to a variety of interpretations, facilitating transcendence in decision-making and activity. Symbols give us meaning that goes beyond the immediacy of our sense impressions. Indeed, power to transcend the context of our lives derives from the symbols with which we identify.

## ADAPTATION

Adaptation is sometimes defined as a process or mechanism which enables us to survive. In evolutionary terms adaptive processes perpetuate the species, whereas maladaptive processes culminate in extinction. Adaptation suggests congruence between specific forms of life and their environment. However, problematic circumstances in the short run may become constructive over time. People migrate to other countries and find it difficult to adjust in a decade; adaptation and assimilation take several generations.

Adaptation is not synonymous with compromise at micro levels of interaction. Giving in to the demands and expectations of others is ultimately a maladaptive process. Adaptation must enhance life, a purpose which goes beyond meeting others' demands. Adaptation is more effective when our action is autonomous and our decision-making deliberate. We do not need merely to accommodate others. Persistent compromise in the negotiations of values with others is maladaptive. Although flexibility in dealing with others is beneficial, self-sacrifice for others' is overly adaptive and self-destructive.

Historically and culturally women have adapted to others without self-consideration or cultivation of an awareness of identity. These overly adaptive modes have enfeebled women, making their relationships and activities problematic. In their central roles as wives and mothers, women frequently nurture spouse and children without valuing their own lives.

Focusing on identity alters women's adaptive patterns. When they act from a self that is centered in their own being, women become freer to act in their own interests and more effective in adapting to broader forces of change.

When we consider evolution and change, we are able to identify patterns of behavior that lead to functional adaptation rather than extinction. However, the primacy of values and ideals in our lives suggests that fulfillment is more necessary to us as direction or goal than is survival itself.

Values influence our views of evolution and self, and identity clarifies purpose in our lives. Goals and ideals transcend our empirical situations. When we act deliberately, becoming a willing participant in evolution, both our human dignity and our animal instincts contribute to our adaptation. Evolution occurs whether we consciously participate in it or not. The quality of our lives is improved though when we act with an awareness of evolution. If we are to live fully, we must respond to life with awareness.

Adaptation is more than survival of the fittest or the triumphs of military strength. These modes of adaptation are possibilities, but they are not optimal or even feasible in the long run because they necessitate the destruction of others. Adaptation can be more altruistic or mutually life-enhancing. One significant characteristic of being human is the capacity to modify some of the influence of instincts. Identity empowerment is a mechanism which allows people to transcend their automatic or reactive behavior and to harness this emotional energy for work towards goals or ideals.

Adaptation by groups may be detrimental to the individual member's fulfillment. In patriarchal societies males have more power and status than females, living longer than females where medical innovations have not reduced mortality at childbirth. Even though women adapt to these social conditions, their continued subordination works against their own interest.

Identity empowerment of women and men reduces maladaptation and facilitates overall adaptation for larger numbers of people. As women become stronger, they express their own real interests. It is only when women see that autonomous adaptation is necessary that they are motivated to change their habitual pattern of centering their lives around the needs of others.

## ASSUMPTIONS

Whether or not we are aware of our beliefs about evolution and change, we all make assumptions about the universe, nature, and human nature. We take for granted that humans have certain basic characteristics and we formulate our expectations through this understanding. Generally we do not question our assumptions about ourselves and the world. The assumptions we make about life help to define the ways in which we live and interact with others. We act according to who or what we believe we are, and what we believe the world to be. In these respects the concept of identity and identity mechanisms are crucial. We change our behavior and activity in substantial ways when we are aware of our self-perception. Identity and self-concept motivate our actions.

A first step in becoming self-aware is to examine our assumptions about ourselves, others, and the universe. On occasion, seeing ourselves within the context of social and natural systems prompts us to address limitations. Thus assumptions about the universe have a distinct impact on definitions of human nature. If we accept scientific theories of evolution, we will be less likely to view or experience human beings as moral creatures. We tend to see ourselves as dominated by instinct and emotion. Evolutionary theorists emphasize the competitive aspects of human nature rather than idealistic characteristics, believing in the essential nonrationality of human behavior.

Other assumptions about behavior may be more closely aligned with religion, such as believing that God is revealed in history. Human nature in this context is perceived as enhanced through learning. These alternative assumptions suggest that human nature is not limited by the expression of animal instincts, but rather that human behavior can be rational and responsible.

We have choices to make in our understanding of evolution and change. We select assumptions which relate directly to our own experiences and meanings. If we uncritically accept others' beliefs, we risk perpetuating unawareness of self. Women need their own definitions of change and evolution. Their behavior flows from their particular interpretations of the universe and life. When they make positive, humane assumptions about themselves, they have greater opportunities for expansive fulfillment.

It is not easy to modify our assumptions, particularly those we have unconsciously accepted. We must make deliberate resolutions about our knowledge and understanding of the universe in order to become the subject rather than object or victim of our beliefs. Our awareness derives from these interpretations.

Although we try to assemble all relevant facts and make reasoned judgments about evolution and change, inferences are ultimately necessary as human minds cannot know or grasp all the pertinent information. We must live with some beliefs about reality, and we label these beliefs evolutionary theory, religion, or political ideology. Some beliefs reflect empirical conditions directly and predict events more accurately than others. Effective belief systems are also sufficiently flexible to adapt to the increasingly complex body of knowledge.

Values permeate our beliefs about reality and the assumptions we make about ourselves, others, and the universe. Values are units of our beliefs. We choose values about life, although in most respects it is easier to use the values internalized from childhood. Our assumptions about the world must express our interests if we are to live fully. Personal or social crises frequently shake the foundations of our beliefs, showing us that we need to change our values and assumptions to survive. If we see destructiveness in the values of our daily lives, we must question and change our assumptions in order to live productively. Makeshift changes in behavior are less effective in problem resolution than modifications or substitutions in our assumptions about life. Identity mechanisms benefit women and strengthen their functioning when they select life values with which to identify. Women who believe bearing children is their sole purpose live differently from women who believe that in addition to bearing children they can achieve goals which contribute directly to society.

## HISTORY

History is a concept and discipline which describes changes through time. Time dimensions are an essential aspect of identity concerns and choices. Based largely on written records, historical methodologies are ill-equipped to gauge the broader scope of evolutionary theory, turning instead to human civilization in the last several thousand years. In recent years, historians have been criticized by feminists for a bias in favor of patriarchal values. For example, political developments are described without references to women, and it is only in relatively contemporary times that historians have collected information about women's lives.

Historians have collected their most detailed data from the last few thousand years to document current changes in society. The data can be used to assess significant influences on and patterns in women's lives. For example, preindustrial conditions are historically more disadvantageous for women, as their options are quite circumscribed. In general, the segregation and subordination of women in a wide range of societies is well-documented by historical research.

Women understand themselves more fully by comparing their experiences across time and historical literacy enables women to defined their destinies more actively. By understanding and acknowledging changes, they can see direction and potential in their lives. Individual lives are far better understood— and self-consciously shaped—if they are viewed as integral to human history. Women effectively seize opportunities for change when they know what their starting point is.

Historical studies suggest the pervasiveness and tenacity of problem conditions for women, and the extent to which restrictions and prohibitions have existed in all times and in all places. Historical research documents that men's interest groups have continuously dominated political systems through their ability to organize themselves effectively around their interests.

Continuities in women's subordination are described in a variety of ways. Historical studies imply that women's limitations are passed from generation to generation, and that these processes affect social organization and interaction. In wartime there is greater acceptance of equality, but after these crises are resolved, conventional beliefs about prosperity pressure women to return to their subordinate statuses.

Women have always been and always will be participants in historical processes. Limitations in women's lives are typical of particular historical periods. As historians have relatively ignored women, women are challenged to rewrite history by collecting new information and by synthesizing fragments of knowledge about women. This contribution modifies the discipline's past and present male-centeredness, allowing women to establish their equality in the human heritage.

Historical precedents do not determine the quality of women's lives, although data show the overwhelming power of the institutional influences women must surmount in order to achieve independence and equality. Studies of discrimination against women in the labor force document other limiting forces in women's lives. However, historical accounts may motivate women to recognize patterns and challenge the sources of their oppression. Women need no longer passively accept positions as victims of social institutions and established trends.

It is understandable that some women may not be able to gather sufficient emotional and physical resources to push themselves through the limitations society places on them as agents of change. Identity mechanisms neutralize many of these difficulties. When identity is empowered, empirical conditions are circumvented or transcended in ways that less informed efforts cannot accomplish. Although obstacles remain, identity clarification allows women to focus on goals rather than on difficulties, thereby becoming more effective and more active participants in historical change and evolution. In this respect, then, identity is both time-specific and eternal. Women act in present circumstances, but move towards lasting goals and ideals that transcend the present.

## GOALS

One of the differences that distinguishes human beings from other creatures is that humans choose goals for their activity. Humans are not necessarily driven by instincts or emotions as are other animals. Humans may opt to move towards their own selected goals or ideals. When we know who we are and have honestly analyzed our present situations, we can articulate objectives and options. Identity awareness is a precondition for defining goals or purposes in our lives. Achieving a deliberately chosen identity imbues our lives with meaning.

Historically most women have neither been in a position to clarify or construct their own identity nor to articulate and select their own goals. They have lacked the necessary autonomy and freedom to do this. Only recently have women been sufficiently in charge of their own lives to be able to plan goals and directions.

Clarification and empowerment of identity may be considered as goals that women select. Identity, however, is less an end in itself than it is a means for fulfillment. We pursue fulfillment and the benefits it brings as ends in themselves.

As more women become educated, their motivation to achieve particular occupational and professional goals increases. Education generates new possibilities, avenues of mobility, and higher goals for women. Whatever the area of study, learning is an important way to broaden horizons. The major part of women's efforts towards increased achievement lies in articulating goals rather than in striving and surmounting obstacles. Goals push women forward, enabling them to surmount obstacles with greater ease than frontal attacks on circumstances.

Our goals may be ideal or practical and mundane. Whatever the case, goals must be taken seriously as representing the basic need for expression. Indeed, without meaningful goals, life is empty. As society evolves, goals evolve. Possibilities come into being that could not be imagined in prior times. Goals can be one of the significant moving forces in history, especially when they articulate religious beliefs or transcendental ideals. For example, Protestantism started a valuing of individual conscience, one of its goals being direct communion with God.

Although goals may be highly personal and unique, they may also be universal. Universal goals embrace crude survival needs as well as needs for full development. Various cultures define fulfillment differently, but life satisfaction is a universal goal. Goals are products of the values we cherish. In times of rapid change, ambiguities in values make goals more difficult to define. Goals tend to reflect the cultural continuities of particular groups and specific periods. In the past, women worked toward goals centered around others. Since these goals were not of women's own creation, they did not bring personal satisfaction. For the first time large numbers of women articulate, sustain, and achieve their own goals.

Goals need not engender competition. We formulate goals for ourselves rather than pursue scarce resources or others' objectives. For example, women and men can choose to work towards more universal, nonmaterial goals. This minimizes competition within society. Nonmaterial goals and ideals fortify our identity. We are our goals, and our fulfillment lies in working toward their accomplishment.

## GENERALIZATIONS AND PROPOSITIONS

Change and evolution are related to concerns of women and identity in a variety of ways. The generalizations that follow establish a context for more specific studies of identity and quality of women's lives.

**1** Our understanding of self and identity depends upon our understanding of change and evolution. That is, we act on the assumptions we make about the universe and human nature.

**2** Identity options are polarized by contrasts in evolutionary and religious beliefs. Human beings are seen as instinct-driven, competitive animals in evolution, or they are conceptualized as moral beings who can transform themselves through learning and religion.

**3** Historical precedents do not circumscribe possibilities of change or determine outcomes. Evolution suggests that new phenomena are produced and that there are quantum leaps in development.

**4** Intensified ambiguities in values in times of rapid change make identity more difficult to clarify.

**5** Historical data are needed to increase our objective understanding of women and identity. Nuances in the repeated patterns of women's segregation and subordination are delineated in historical research.

**6** Perceptions of change and evolution are major subjective influences on women's lives, and shape both identity and behavior.

**7** Selecting goals is an effective mechanism for achieving long-range adaptation in evolutionary processes.

Current opportunities for women to empower identity depend on contemporary structures in their lives. The impact of change and evolution on women and identity is assessed in the following propositions.

**1** One of the most crucial levels of understanding self and others consists of the assumptions we make about the nature of human nature and the nature of the universe. These assumptions must be questioned or changed as a prerequisite for changing identity.

2   Identity is a mechanism that brings about the more effective adaptation of women to their environment. Identity promotes women's life satisfaction and contributions to society.

3   Goals are mechanisms which allow women to transcend or neutralize the power of institutional structures blocking their opportunities.

4   Our assumptions and goals are eventually tested by reality. Beliefs that are too far removed from empirical conditions are counterproductive and ultimately destructive for self and others.

5   A fuller understanding of evolutionary change enables women to be more active participants in evolution.

6   Women who align their identities with historical circumstances have a greater impact on society and social change than women who establish identities unrelated to historical conditions.

7   The deliberate selection of meaningful goals enhances the quality of life of women by opening possibilities other than automatic reaction to others and circumstances. Choices make deviations from the norm possible.

Chapter 7

# Commitment

In order to live fully we need purpose and direction in our activities. Random, nondeliberate action is experienced as meaningless. Patterning in our responses to situations is necessary for personal and social satisfaction.

We create our own purposes and directions through myriad decisions. Our decisions flow from the commitments we make according to our perceived purposes and directions. When we make deliberate commitments and follow through with action, we function beyond survival levels of existence. Our commitments express our deepest values and sometimes require vision beyond our everyday existence. By transcending empirical conditions we move towards satisfaction and fulfillment, and in the process meet our survival needs.

Only when we are aware of available options can our decisions be responsible in the broad context of change. Our personal milieus are connected to public domains, and we need to acknowledge this as our focus for attention.

In a time of increasing opportunities and possibilities, it is unenlightened to choose merely to repeat traditional patterns of behavior without assessing alternatives. We have the responsibility to create new pathways. This is life. Flexibility, change, and living fully require new modes of adaptation. For women especially, business cannot be conducted as usual.

Even opting for traditional roles after a careful consideration of options increases purpose and meaning, as more deliberate decision-making transforms attitudes and activity into conscious acts. Blind faith and unquestioning attitudes must be modified or thrust aside if our lives are to be transformed.

Commitments are a consequence and culmination of our values. We cannot make a full commitment to a career or marriage unless we value work or companionship. If we change our values, we must change our commitments.

Our most effective commitments are not rigid but flexible and durable. Closed, narrow commitments prove brittle under the stresses of daily life. In order to sustain us over time, patterns of values in our commitments must tolerate change.

Breathing space in our commitments is necessary for their meaningful fulfillment, for life itself. We do not make self-contained, ultimate decisions at specific points in time. Rather, we participate in a sequence or flow of commitments. Our commitments must be fluid; restrictive commitments cannot sustain our humanity.

Our commitments shape the ways in which we respond to situations. Our actions in specific circumstances are defined by our basic values. The substance of our values dictates whether responses will be creative and expansive or restrictive and destructive. In the pursuit of goals, our commitments are experienced as stable and even permanent. Commitments imply a conscious and deliberate selection of goals and an expression of values. We empower ourselves by choosing our values and commitments. When we know the foundation on which our values are built, we become more able to use reason and our other faculties in our own interests and others' interests. We clarify and confirm our view of ourselves and our lives through our commitments. We free ourselves of restrictions and harness our energies more effectively when our decisions are formulated as commitments.

Women embody more meaning in their lives by considering the broader picture of their circumstances and choices. Meaning also derives from their making efforts to respond to opportunities to their advantage and to the advantage of other women. They need to become aware of their shared experiences before they are able to act in concert and move beyond their current level of self-awareness.

Cultivating an awareness of one's inner self increases awareness of spirit and capacity to transcend empirical reality. Moral power and spiritual equality support, motivate, and guide all activities. Our inner resources give us the strength to face and deal with the most intolerable conditions.

Our commitments structure patterns in social interaction. Women assume effective leadership positions by exerting the values which are most real to them. Society's resistance to changing traditional feminine values is predictable, but this can be tempered by understanding and persistence. In this way alternative values are infiltrated into the mainstream.

A patriarchal society is imbalanced and destructive to large proportions of the population. The common good can only develop through a harmonization of masculine and feminine values. Narrow, specific gender interests must give way to broader definitions of gender before fulfillment can occur. Current social breakdown cannot be relieved or remedied through expressing divisive patriarchal values. Productive change results from transitions which incorporate an increased proportion of feminine values, with a tolerance for both female and male values. Community is an ideal for which we can strive with self-respect. Competition cannot produce the good that can only be accomplished through cooperation.

Values and commitments are not impersonal social products. They are the essence of our being and identity. We empower ourselves by knowing and realizing these connections between the whole and the part, between society and ourselves. We are able to flow with constructive, life-enhancing forces when we empower our identities with chosen values and broadened commitments.

## PURPOSE

Identity merges with purpose in the commitments we make. It is through our commitments that we discover who we are, who we have been, and who we can be.

Identity embodies our deepest meanings. When we look at the world with awareness and knowledge of identity, we see new ways in which we can be and act. Value choices in identity predispose us to express ourselves in related commitments. Our fullest and most meaningful expressions of self grow out of these commitments. Identity is empowered when we act in accordance with our own interests rather than react to others' interests. Regardless of others' demands upon us, we must center ourselves in our own identity and commitments.

Women need to define their own purpose, not derive purpose from traditional patriarchal values. Commitments are goal-directed decisions and activities. Identity is increasingly empowered as women select goals that contribute to the common good more directly. A basic and necessary purpose for both women and men is to act in ways which sustain or add to the welfare of the human community.

Commitments are patterned by decisions and purpose; purposes underlie our decisions and commitments. Purpose extends self, including both what we know of ourselves and what we deliberately choose as ours. Identity is a starting point for commitments that express purpose in our lives.

Some of our purposes are more crucial to our identity than others. In order to be effective and efficient, it is important to become single-minded about having a central purpose and commitments. Another way to think of this process is to see identity and commitments as linked to a primary goal, aim, or ideal. For example, a goal to contribute to knowledge brings with it a variety of specific value choices, decisions, and commitments. Commitments must be sufficiently flexible to enable individuals to grow and strengthen self through interaction. Our negotiations and contracts with others need to be reaffirmed or remade in the midst of changing circumstances. Our purposes may remain remarkably stable over long periods of time, but the means we choose to express purpose may shift or be modified, particularly in periods of rapid change.

Thus, purpose reinforces human dignity and structures the human condition. Although all animals have dignity, only human beings reflect upon their lives and make choices to express purpose. Commitments and purpose relate to both short and long time periods. Timing is a significant element in the coherence and consistency of commitments and purpose. In order for identity to be strong, we must choose commitments that will promote inner harmony and consistency. Coherence in identity and commitments expresses a flow of life energy that affects others in constructive rather than destructive ways. One of our purposes is to find a specific purpose of our own which will enhance this flow of life and outpouring of energy.

## DIRECTION

Direction can be thought of as an extension of identity and purpose. We cannot always define direction in our lives, but we do move in some direction, our awareness or desire notwithstanding. Our direction may be counterproductive to our intentions or neutralized by random and purposeless action. When direction is clear, guided by purpose and fueled by a clear and deliberate sense of identity, activity is more likely to have an effective impact on others.

The plotting of direction in our lives from past events gives a substantive base to our reflections about identity and commitments. We understand ourselves more fully when we make efforts to discern past and present directions in our lives. Direction is frequently created more from our value choices and related goals than by inner efforts or striving.

Direction in women's lives is customarily imposed by others rather than self-generated. Women do not have many socially acceptable options available to them, and their choices are largely unidirectional. Reacting to pressure from social expectations such as marriage and parenthood, women move towards integration with traditional patriarchal values. Repetitions and restrictions in direction are passed from mother to daughter through many generations.

Life is expansive, and women's newly discovered directions take them into the broadest social arenas. Commitments to careers and other activities allow women to interact in contexts other than the traditional domains of family and religion. Women also exert greater authority in their own families, as well as move from devotional congregant roles to leadership in organized religion.

Thus, identity implies direction in life, and getting to know one's values facilitates the discovery of a latent direction. Having direction is liberating, especially for women, as direction transcends everyday routines. It is through direction that women become sufficiently motivated to neutralize or break through their entrapments in patriarchal societies.

Direction helps us to synthesize and give meaning to our commitments over time. We can only get to where we want to go when we have a clear starting point as well as a specific goal. Goals alone are not enough. To move forward we must examine past decisions and retrace past directions in order to know where we have come from and what our choices are.

Crises generally disrupt our plans and wreak havoc with our emotions, making our lives seem without purpose and direction. More constructively, crises can be thought of as turning points and opportunities to reevaluate identity and direction. These shifts in our beliefs prompt us to develop a new self-image and survival tactics. Crises frequently generate dramatic changes in our lives—we may decide upon a new career or develop our talents in a particular direction for a decade or more.

Women's new directions, such as living according to their own interests, may disrupt commitments and relationships. Overall direction, like the continued development of their potential, is of paramount importance. Establishing a meaningful direction for ourselves must be one of our highest priorities since it influences all of our value choices and decision-making. Our commitments express our direction, but there are times when direction overtakes our current commitments and relationships, leading us to establish new ones.

Whatever our direction, we need to stay alert to the present and take opportunities that are in our interest. Women cannot allow nostalgia, sentiment, and tradition to draw them back into a past which restricts their lives. On the other hand, women cannot live only for the future. They must be rooted in the present, and be aware of current trends and events in order to proceed effectively towards a promising future.

Women remain vulnerable to others' directions, especially since obedience and loyalty are traditional women's values in patriarchal societies. Women must be vigilant to ensure that they direct their own lives. When they put a premium on doing what others request, they jeopardize their ability to achieve their own goals, define their own purposes, and direct their own lives. Direction in living characterizes those who feel fulfilled and achieve a great deal. Accomplishment is frequently precipitated by a sense of being guided or inwardly led to our goals.

If we cannot discern direction in our lives, we should trust life and move on to our next task. Frequently it is only in retrospect that we can discover our direction, although we may be aware of our choices and actions. We can have confidence that identity will guide us in diverse ways towards more meaning.

## PATTERNS

Patterns in individual and social commitments, values, and behavior can be identified. The patterns we establish do not exist in isolation, but are interconnected with those of others. Patterns in commitments and values exist whether or not individuals are aware of them. It is difficult to identify specific patterns because they move along time lines in unfamiliar ways. Although patterns are repeated, some behavior is ambiguous. Patterns in commitments and values give order to interpersonal behavior. Priorities and consistencies underlie our behavior at all times.

Patterns exist at invisible levels of human connectedness and in observable negotiations. For example, we are often quite visibly more loyal to ancestors and deceased relatives than to our contemporaries. Patterns in lifetime commitments, such as marriage or career, generally express our values clearly. We approach our spouses or colleagues with characteristic styles of communication, and our priorities extend into action. Values generate patterns of behavior and commitments.

There is a basic orderliness in our psychic, interpersonal, and behavioral commitments. Although we may never be able to understand all aspects of the subjective and objective orders of our lives, some suppositions are suggested by facts.

Identity enables us to predict our own and others' responses. Patterns in our commitments derive directly from identity, the internalized order in our values. If we change the order of our values or the substance of the values with which we identify, patterns in our behavior shift to correlate with our new values or the new order of our values.

Patterned values underlie different modes of conformity and are characterized by narrower, more rigid values than deviancy. Unlike modern values, traditional values have continuities. Traditional values, such as authority, have a long history and institutional legitimation. Modern values are more varied and innovative than traditional values. Modern values generate new, diverse patterns in commitments, whereas traditional values are characterized by uninterrupted repetitions of patterns.

Commitments are established, maintained, narrowed, stretched, or broken. They are a starting point of adaptation through behavior and a foundation for patterned responses. Patterns in commitment behavior range from conflict to harmony, conflict manifesting more distinctive patterns. Conflict makes us aware of our choices, revealing new options we might not otherwise have discovered. We have choices in establishing our order of values in identity, and patterned behavior flows from the priorities we establish.

Our commitments focus on ourselves as well as on other people. Traditionally women have made most of their commitments to others rather than to themselves. Feminists have pointed out women's self-destruction and self-depletion through overcommitment to family members. The clarity and intensity in women's commitments to others means that they lose themselves through focusing on duties and obligations. Women live vicariously when they derive purpose solely through loyalty and dedication. Their challenge is to transform commitments to others into commitments to themselves. Influencing priorities in all decision-making, commitments form the foundation of patterns in behavior. Their orderliness derives from the values with which women identify.

Historically, women's commitments relate to narrower domains than men's. Women have been limited to being family caretakers or models of religious devotion. Men's commitments, by contrast, contain much broader patterns of commitments, such as political representation and career advancement. Also, whereas women's patterns confine them to the same areas throughout their lives, men achieve mobility through changing the objects and range of their commitments. Men have also sustained openness in their patterns by opportunities for personal and professional development. This openness contrasts with the rigidity and closed qualities of patterns in women's commitments, such as responsibility for caring for an aging parent until death.

## ACTION

Identity is an alignment of values in hierarchies which add meaning to our lives. This ordering relates in some way to values conventionally associated with gender.

Our awareness of identity and values is not an intellectual exercise. Values are an emotional aspect of our being and are among the most intractable aspects of human nature. In some respects identity is the most durable but also the most vulnerable center of our being. Values are inextricable components of social relations—interaction is not possible without some shared values.

Values orient our behavior, whether or not we act with deliberation and choice. One of the clearest manifestations of our values and behavior is the series of commitments we undertake during our lives. If we seek truth or reality, for example, we value knowledge and intellectual pursuits in our quest.

Behavior is movement towards meeting needs such as nourishment or companionship. Action is more deliberate than behavior, flowing from enlightened being or reflective modes of consciousness. We make our most meaningful commitments when we give thought to them, that is, when we are fully aware of the scope and consequences of our action.

Action is a prerequisite of living fully, and our commitments evolve from deliberate action. Commitments form a foundation for structured action. Even spontaneous, unplanned activity is directly related to our commitments. We participate in leisure activities which flow from social status or family role. If we reorder our values through loosening class loyalties or family obligations, our commitments and activity also change.

Historically women have been conditioned to respond to others' actions rather than to act autonomously. As a result of this passivity women have fewer but more intense commitments than men, their mission being to serve and support family members, or to labor to meet subsistence needs. A significant way out of this entrapment is for women to give more attention to their action, trying to move in the direction of their own interests rather than to react to others' demands or expectations. Through action women develop their potential and come into what is rightfully theirs. Living fully and being fulfilled are accomplished only when activity flows from women's commitments to develop their own interests.

Historical and cross-cultural research suggests that women's work demands more time and energy than men's, though this labor has been concentrated in limited milieus such as the family. Traditionally, women's relationship networks are immediate community members, with little possibility of moving beyond these restricted circles. Their labor entrenches them in passive modes in relation to the wider society.

Action breaks cycles of reactivity and automatic behavior. When women act from conditioning rather than awareness, their action is programmed. When they think their action through according to their own interests, they act more fully. Awareness followed by enlightened action interrupts and disrupts chains of emotional reactivity, creating openings and possibilities for women to move into new active responses.

A significant chain of behavior is the repetition among the intergenerational bonds of grandmothers, mothers, and daughters. Behavior passed from generation to generation can be broken, however, and such disruption has long-term constructive consequences. Although women tend to marry and bear children in similar patterns in several generations, as successive generations realize increased degrees of freedom through deliberate action, a future of freedom for women is assured.

Commitment is a necessary activity. Deliberate action can only flow from decisions and established priorities. When women have a clear idea of who they are, they structure commitments in their own interests and to enhance their lives and others' lives. Women's identity needs to be expressed in action so they can live fully. Action is essential for a more complete expression of life.

## RESPONSIBILITY

Responsibility is a moral concept based on the assumption that human beings have choices. Some choices are viewed as being more worthy or appropriate than others. Responsibility implies a sense of obligation or duty to act in specific normatively defined ways—to behave so one meets with the approval of mainstream society.

Responsibility suggests mission in life. We exist to achieve some purpose. Another assumption about responsibility is that there is a moral imperative that dictates decisions conducive to accomplishing our purpose.

Responsibility is also our acceptance of the challenge to make the most of our lives. Depending on our view of the world or humanity, we understand ourselves to have potential for accomplishment. Even though there is much evidence of human frailty, as long as people make monumental contributions to civilization, it is conceivable that these energies and powers are available to all—to those who make such requests and demands from life, existence, or themselves.

Responsibility includes our acceptance of our own uniqueness and the special circumstances of our lives. When we acknowledge who and where we are, we move away from conformity as an end in itself. We live more authentically by acting with interest and contributing to the collective good. As women traditionally denied their own interests, they consequently made only a narrow range of contributions to society. When women learn to trust themselves and identify with power rather than passivity, they move into less familiar territories with confidence, and lead more fulfilling lives. This expansive mode of living generates a broad range of contributions to the collective good.

We may equate fulfillment with responsibility. If we believe that people are entitled to be fulfilled by virtue of being human, it is our responsibility to act in ways that lead towards our fulfillment. We share responsibility to make the world as good as possible. We cannot transform human nature or many of the givens of our social conditions, but we can identify ourselves as our strongest selves, transmitting that power to coming generations. We define our responsibility as women by continuing to develop our potential, as our foremothers did or tried to do. The call of responsibility to attend to and accomplish this task galvanizes women to devote their energies to these goals single-mindedly.

Our responsibility rests primarily in our ability to make choices. We need to delineate options and make decisions in accordance with our long-range objectives, and cannot afford to succumb to short-range distractions or pressures. Our responsibility is to move towards ideals rather than makeshift compromises. When we do not accept these challenges our decisions are irresponsible, even if we are not yet aware of our full range of choices.

Traditionally, women have been coerced to accept others' definitions of situations. They have not been given socially acceptable options beyond strict conformity to patriarchal values. Women who reject traditional female roles have been stigmatized as deviants rather than viewed as innovators or pioneers carving out additional options and possibilities. Women have a primary responsibility to be true to themselves and to assist other women in that task. Identity awareness and identity empowerment are mechanisms that contribute towards this ideal. If women change their direction in life, the foundation of society is transformed. Relationships and social structures become more balanced, life satisfaction being increased for all. Women's commitments and behavior generate new patterns of gender egalitarianism and individual and social fulfillment.

It is women's responsibility to enter into expansive commitments seriously. We cannot live interdependent lives without commitments, and we must act responsibly in order to meet our commitments. Our lives are limited by our basic needs, but we are not defined or determined by these needs. Whereas we need to have commitments in our lies, our freedom lies in choosing commitments which flow directly from our own interests and values.

## FULFILLMENT

Fulfillment makes our lives whole and complete. Women can only be fulfilled through chosen commitments. They need to be fulfilled, or to be working towards fulfillment, in order to survive through long periods. Fulfillment transcends all our goals. We express ourselves best when we aim to develop our potential and make contributions to the collective good.

Women have not been taught or shown how to fulfill themselves. Women have been conditioned to allow or encourage others to be fulfilled. Women's nurturing and supportive roles facilitate the development of children, parents, and men, but not of themselves. Such self-sacrificing activities cannot honor the fullness of life because women cannot express themselves completely through caretaking. Others' demands exert coercive influences on women, often persuading them to sacrifice their interests. This is too high a price for women to pay, and too high a price for those for whom their sacrifices are made since they also suffer from women's lack of fulfillment.

Fulfillment must be envisioned before it can come into being. All members of a collective—regardless of gender, race, or status—need to be fulfilled so that each can function effectively.

Commitments bring substance and specificity to our daily routines. We have to deal with reality in particular ways and pay attention to detail when we live out our commitments. Commitments may be restrictive, such as domestic roles, or expansive, such as career contributions, but only our most expansive and meaningful commitments result in fulfillment. When women are aware of these differences, they are better able to act in their own interests. If women persist in sacrificing themselves to others without pursuing or even denying their own fulfillment, society will remain unbalanced, perpetuating restrictions in both women's and men's lives.

Women can help each other work towards their own fulfillment. Major commitments they make aid this process. They serve as models of fulfillment for other women, and assist in the development of their potential.

Fulfillment accompanies the establishment of purpose and direction in our lives. It results from life-enhancing commitments which provide opportunities for growth and empowerment. Responsible action flows from commitments to collective well-being and fulfillment.

Fulfillment is derived from identity awareness and related action. It does not happen by chance. We make choices that lead to fulfillment or dissatisfaction. Values are guides in the choices we make, and they anchor us in a world of change. We negotiate values with others so that our animal dependencies do not overwhelm us.

We move towards fulfillment through modes of belonging. We are not fulfilled in isolation, but only through others. We examine change and broader evolutionary processes so that we can achieve fulfillment by acting in harmony with our own life forces. Repression and suppression do not give us the freedom we need to participate in change and evolution.

We develop "religions" of fulfillment by ordering our most important values into a meaningful hierarchy. Our beliefs are constructed from our values, and it is our most significant values that form the core and substance of our fulfillment.

Feminist gains are strengthened and promoted through women's efforts towards fulfillment. Women's goal-directed activity increases possibilities for the fulfillment of all, not just women themselves. Fulfillment is necessary for the balance of individual women and society as a whole. Women choose to deviate by selecting their own values as the core of their lives rather than to conform by reacting to others' demands and pressures.

Women choose modern values so they can be increasingly fulfilled. Traditional values may also be selected. New combinations of traditional values may provide sufficient flexibility for innovative action by women. Our crises and conflicts are lived with more comfortably when we see that they move us towards fulfillment. Our lives are more predictably enjoyable when we aim for fulfillment through commitments.

Identity is the source of our intentions for fulfillment. Identity is our guide for making commitments. New levels of being emerge as we develop our potential and bring our fulfillment into the present rather than think of it as a tentative possibility for the future.

The scope of our fulfillment is limited only by evolutionary parameters of life. Human laws and norms can be changed, whereas natural laws are relatively immutable. Strong women have established precedents for us to follow and extend. Women are tenacious and persevering, just as those who have gone before them in their quests for fulfillment.

## GENERALIZATIONS AND PROPOSITIONS

Complexities in human beings are easily oversimplified and distorted by generalizations and propositions. The intent of the following summary statements is to single out some of the most basic patterns and tendencies in interaction, and to suggest guides for interpretation and understanding.

Unless women cultivate more effective ways to understand their lives, they will remain vulnerable to all the vicissitudes and restrictions of their historical and contemporary experiences. They can only forge more expansive life-enhancing patterns of living and fulfillment by selecting their commitments with increased awareness.

These generalizations about women, identity, and commitment can be made.

**1**  To the extent that women increase their awareness of their identity and commitment, purpose, direction, and fulfillment will be increased.

**2**  Commitment is an active component of identity. When identity is clarified, commitments become more deliberate and meaningful.

**3**  Commitment to realize women's most important values in action gives direction and stability in times of rapid change.

**4**  Women's roles are redefined and autonomy increased by rearranging, decreasing, or increasing their commitments.

**5**  Women enter into the flow of life more fully by selecting goals of their choice rather than by reacting to others' demands and expectations.

**6**  Women belong to each other and to the human race in more viable ways when the bonds of their commitments are based on their own real interests. Women's interests are essential to society, and can be expressed fully only through commitments.

**7**  Chosen commitments allow women to be more active participants in evolutionary processes.

More specific propositions are derived from these generalizations and connections between women, identity, and commitment.

**1**  Identity and commitment are powerful change mechanisms. To the extent that women choose more modern, autonomous values as bases of identity and commitment, everyone's lives are enhanced.

**2**  When identity and commitments are expansive, women are better able to transcend restrictions and limitations in their traditional roles.

**3**  The most enduring commitments are flexible, related to both self-interests and the interests of society. Commitments also need to be flexible to withstand social pressures.

**4** Commitments stabilize individuals and society by establishing particular patterns of interaction and postures in negotiations of values.

**5** Personal and social fulfillment result from planned commitments. Commitments are predictably and inextricably related to identity.

**6** We create and sustain our freedom through choosing values for identity and commitment. Cultivated freedom is real and deep.

**7** Commitments are necessary for fulfillment, which itself is necessary for survival. Women must care enough about themselves and other women so that they can move from half-living to fulfillment.

# Chapter 8

# Success

Though success can be defined in innumerable ways, socioeconomic status is typically used as the measure. Gender or ethnic stereotypes define alternative styles of success. Success can also be measured in biological terms. Staying alive and active receives some acclaim in old age. Success, health, and wholeness are ways people lead satisfying lives.

Success for women traditionally means adapting to others' needs and demands. Historically, a successful woman was one who put her husband and children before herself, being unaware that her own needs could or should be met. Success for women was conforming to patriarchal norms and expectations that restricted them.

Success for men is closely tied to society's economic rewards for work. Historically, men's work received payment, the accumulation of economic assets being regarded as a key indicator of their success. In order to achieve advancement in work, men compete with each other for authority, power, and scarce resources. It is essential for men to perform competitively in order to be successful.

More androgynous definitions of success are needed before we can move to more egalitarian relations between women and men. New patterns of interaction are initiated more effectively if the success both women and men enjoy is recognized and valued. New modes of success can decrease segregation and inequalities between women and men.

Successful people tend to be at peace with themselves. They are whole and complete in their accomplishments, and they enjoy life by balancing work and play as well as family and individual pursuits. Successful people have meaningful goals, working towards them gradually, effectively, and purposefully. They are tolerant of others and support their efforts to make the most of themselves. Success is incompatible with the oversacrifice of self or destructive behavior.

Ideas and thoughts are important. Women cannot claim more humane standards until they clarify their self-image and objectives. Before they can be successful, women need to see success for what it has long been—a way to receive others' recognition and to be fulfilled.

Success includes both autonomy and conformity. Whatever our goals, human beings need each other. We must conform in order to accomplish tasks and sustain energy. Our unique contributions to society are developed only through self-knowledge. Commitments and goals must be meaningful if we are to be successful in accomplishing them.

The need for success gives women and men opportunities to consider new models. If we are to relate differently, we must become new people. We cannot revert to traditional, segregated models and standards because they do not work towards the development of potential and freedom, especially not for women.

The world is changing rapidly, and increasing numbers of people are aware of their value choices through human rights issues and other social movements. Identity choices generate new standards for success. Education and awareness enable us to see and become the kind of person we want to be. Women cannot merely emulate men in their success styles, nor can men emulate women through their standards. Mechanical imitation is not satisfying. We must become ourselves in this new world, and cultivate tolerance for each other. It is only when we decide to pursue our real interests that this transformation is possible.

## DIMENSIONS OF SUCCESS

Success is multifaceted and experienced in different degrees. Different components of success need to be considered in order to get a clearer and fuller understanding of its nature. In Western society, accumulated scarce resources are considered synonymous with success. As such, success is still largely the privilege of men who inherit wealth or work for remuneration. Women are rarely allowed means of their own except through family inheritance. Today, however, increasing proportions of women are working out of the home, becoming more independent and self-sufficient in their own right.

Material success is transient. High incomes and multiple possessions may not be enjoyed since pressures to spend money in conventional ways frequently run counter to personal preferences. Within these various traditional connotations, success has moral implications. Standards of success and goodness are generally taken to be synonymous with traditional norms and expectations. Pioneering women and men who are trying to live in new and more satisfying ways are seen as deviants more often than not. Success has meant conforming to established patterns of behavior.

Subcultures or ethnic groups may have ranges of values that differ from mainstream society. There are few universal standards of success and many nuances of success derive from within particular subcultures. Control of emotion and expression of emotion are viewed as both success and failure by different cultural and ethnic groups. Men view control of emotion as successful, and women define goodness or success as expressing sentiments such as love.

Standards of success vary at different stages of the life cycle. What we consider success in youth may no longer connote success in old age. The varied explorations of different life-styles among young adults is not considered appropriate later in life. Family demands and work responsibilities change depending on our age, and success in middle-age or older ages may sometimes be realized more by maintaining our positions than by striving for additional achievements. Living productively and staying alive are significant dimensions of success.

Success implies the exercise of autonomy as well as the ability to make responsible choices from available options. In this way success is a state of being or process which is distinct from being a victim of circumstances. Activity rather than passivity characterizes success. Where success does not mean unquestioning conformity to others' standards, accomplishment contributes to well-being.

Success is both universal and particular, including shared experiences as well as unique characteristics. Ideally we find our own niches through socially approved routes of relating to others. Our successful contributions reflect our personal values and identity more than broad-based social expectations. Success moves us beyond demands and needs so that we respond and act outside our prescribed roles.

Success needs to be sustained, whatever dimensions or emphases are of most interest to us. Although throughout history women's success comes from conformity to tradition, a wider variety of success is available to women today. Awareness of identity facilitates setting a course for success in our lives. Others' criticism of our success is inevitable, however, and women need each other's support in order to perpetuate their new models and styles of success.

## WHOLENESS

No one is successful without consciously experiencing and expressing themselves as a whole person. The integration of different aspects of self is important for accomplishing and sustaining successful being and doing. Wholeness is
the balance, harmony, and order that result from conscious decisions to behave
in certain ways in our interaction. If we are to be successful, we must enter into
our own lives and commitments fully.

Conventional models of relationships assert that women and men are com-
plementary, thereby encouraging institutional inequalities. A female-male relationship is thought of as being made up of two halves, rather than two wholes,
one half needing the other. Historically women's lives have been partial and
fragmented. Women are expected to thrive in the shadow of men. They are
referred to as the "better" half of a couple, but this is a demeaning expression
suggesting that neither women nor men are whole in their own right. This
concept does not work because it negates the possibility of each person living
fully and autonomously. Everyone must assume full responsibility as a whole
person in order to have personal and social success. It is through wholeness and
full participation that we avoid failure and achieve success.

We experience failure and lack of satisfaction to the extent that we fragment
and compartmentalize our lives. The external manifestations of success, such as
having the right kind of job or clothes, have some importance but cannot be a
foundation for our lives. Priorities based on external measures of success are
ultimately dissatisfying and fragmenting. Full success calls forth our deepest
sense of integrity and our capacity to make deliberate and meaningful choices of
values.

An examination of all the facts of our lives is one way to enhance our
wholeness and become more alive and successful. Women experience wholeness and increase the probability of their success to the extent that they cultivate
habits of reflection about their responses to others. Examining our actions
broadens our perspective on the present by increasing our objectivity about
ourselves and our possibilities.

Role expectations further fragment women's lives. In modern times, for
example, women compartmentalize their roles into domestic and professional
activities in order to function effectively. Some expectations present women
with incompatible differences and conflicts. Being successful as a mother and as
a professional creates stressful demands on women's time and energy, as well as
conflicts in their ideals.

By becoming whole, women consolidate their energies and resources. They
are creative and successful in their syntheses of life. Attentiveness to all their
needs, wants, and responsibilities enables them to emerge from a state of half-
living. Women's healing and empowerment are achieved through multifaceted

interaction in society. The degree to which they maintain their wholeness in personal and public milieus is the true measure of their success.

## NEW MODES OF SUCCESS

Women's challenge is to redefine success according to their own real interests. To work effectively towards new goals and new ideals, they must support and accept each other in their mutual efforts to realize success on their own terms. Without such teamwork, women's progress towards freer modes of success will be slowed and impaired.

Women transcend narrow, restricted models of traditional success by identifying with life-enhancing values. Motivation to move beyond their inherited role expectations is increased through choosing their own values. Identity empowerment increases women's awareness of opportunities for creative action and more constructive adaptation.

New patterns of success for women generally precipitate others' resistance and pressure to return to more established ways of doing things. Thus, it takes great courage and fortitude for women to step outside of traditional roles and sustain a new direction in their lives. Clinical data suggest that it is not so much fear of failure that inhibits freedom of action for women, but rather fear of losing the acceptance and support of those nearest and dearest to them. Their verbal support notwithstanding, those emotionally closest to women generally cannot live comfortably in these changing dependency patterns when women decide to pioneer in personal and professional activities. Consciously or not, husbands and children may sabotage women's plans and activities, or pressure them to conform to their prior roles.

Each woman is a pioneer in establishing new social norms of success for women. There are some models for women to emulate or imitate, but in times of rapid social change it is necessary for women to be versatile, experimenting with different ways to bring meaning and fulfillment to their lives. This may mean that a woman spends a lifetime working towards success without receiving public recognition or even acceptance for her efforts.

Women's initiative in new modes of success has its most immediate impact on small milieus. Different activities and expectations are most fully experienced within families. One woman's changes in a family brings about changes for other family members, particularly for younger generations of women. Although clinical data show that relatives tend to be more demanding than friends, it is in this context that real change for women must be accomplished if they are to withstand and overcome day-to-day restrictions and pressures in their lives.

Perhaps the most difficult task for women who are pursuing new styles of success is to balance their family and professional responsibilities. Continuing inequities in the division of labor perpetuate women's habitual assumption of homemaking and child-rearing responsibilities when they have full-time work out of the home. Women will be overwhelmed by these demands and expectations unless they share family and home responsibilities with men or other women.

Women's work outside the home has many benefits for children. Youngsters see their mothers' competence in dealing with the outside world as well as family matters, and they find more meaning in their lives by learning that women pursue activities in addition to family roles. A mother who works outside the home opens doors for her children to follow her example.

## IDEAL AND PRACTICALITY

Ideals related to women, particularly those that serve to keep them in subordinate positions by maintaining inequalities and limiting their opportunities, have been generated and perpetuated by both women and men. By restricting socially acceptable areas for women's action, expectations have confined them to domestic and religious or moral domains.

Traditional ideals support the status quo of hierarchically ordered families based on male authority. Patriarchal values within families are extended into society. Cross-cultural research shows that women are excluded from decision-making within families and most social settings. A rationale given for patriarchal ideals is that women need to be protected and shielded from life's vicissitudes by men. However, patriarchal ideals in practice impair women's growth and development, suffocating their spontaneity and urge towards fulfillment.

Patriarchal ideals have more practical advantages for men than for women. The ideal of occupational achievement for men increases their educational and professional opportunities. The restrictions men place on women increase men's latitude. Male supremacy and female subordination become values in their own right within the context of patriarchal ideals, and these values enable men to make more positive contributions to society than women can.

Historically, women are responsible for the practical details of subsistence needs and child-rearing. Women's duties in these areas are strongly influenced by patriarchal ideals rather than their own interests. In recent years more women discern the need for ideals that increase their effectiveness in articulating and achieving goals and objectives which go beyond their domestic roles. When women identify with ideals of autonomy rather than subordination, they transform their behavior. New ideals provide women with new views of the world, of themselves, and of others.

In order to be more successful on their own terms, women must identify and select ideals to empower and enhance their lives. An ideal of action rather than passivity moves women towards fulfillment, at the same time alleviating the drudgery of routine chores. When ideals reflect women's real interests, they have practical consequences for both women and men.

New ideals for women's success have specific advantages. Clinical data suggest that conformity to others' demands or expectations is not beneficial to women's well-being, and that achievement of personally selected goals significantly improves the quality of women's lives. Increased satisfaction from daily activities follows a broadened range of ideals for women. The ultimate implication of these interdependent influences is that our supreme ideal or value transforms the nature of our experiences. When we try to articulate our primary values and ideals, we become more aware of ways in which our attitudes and orientation transform our perceptions and experiences.

## SOCIAL SUCCESS

Among a host of other activities, dating the right kinds of men or working for charitable organizations indicates success for middle-class and upper-class women. Women have traditionally used marriage as an avenue of social mobility. Social success is marriage to a man of superior social status.

Social success for women needs new connotations so that they can enhance their lives. Social success can be redefined to include activities making direct contributions to improving society. Women's talents are needed in the mainstream of society as well as in families, and social success must include activities in both areas.

Social success for women today is often synonymous with professional achievement. If women's professional achievements are services aimed at the common good, their impact is social rather than merely individual. Ideally, women's achievements are cooperative rather than competitive ventures, characterized by new patterns of interaction based on women's values.

Women eliminate their dependency on men by concentrating on remunerated work efforts. When they take themselves seriously as whole human beings, women make more effective and substantial contributions. This enlargement of women's lives changes their activity in society, and increases their autonomy and strength within their families. Women enjoy parenting more, and are more effective as parents and wives, when they develop their potential than if their lives remain circumscribed by domestic and family responsibilities.

Social success includes cultivating a sense of humor. This gives women greater objectivity about themselves and greater detachment from male values. All too often conventional humor belittles women. Instead of accepting humor that reinforces the objectification of women as sex objects or possessions, women free themselves by seeing life for what it is, and by emphasizing human strengths and equality.

Women's success can also be described in terms of a religious or spiritual search and expression. Although denominational structures may impede changes for women, religious or spiritual values can add meaning to women's lives as sources of identity and empowerment. Religious or spiritual values

strengthen and support women's quest for deeper understanding and more effective participation or contribution by increasing their motivation to honor
their innate spiritual equality.

Most religious traditions subordinate women to men. Women transcend
some of these limitations by believing that they are equal members of a specific
religious or spiritual heritage. Women's understanding of themselves is a primary influence in their motivation and behavior. When women believe they
have equal access to the sacred, they are empowered and more effective in goal-
setting and behavior. Equality must be claimed and made one's own through
identity and commitments.

If women are unable to find equality through established denominations
and sects, they can select parts of different religious traditions as their own
source of inspiration and motivation. An eclectic approach to religion tends to
be more privatized than social, and may not include sharing community with
others. This source of inspiration and social success is less visible than community participation in specific religious groups.

Women can opt to concentrate on their own spiritual growth and development. Though individual in nature, this approach to the sacred has social consequences. Personal reflection, contemplation, or meditation on the powers of the
universe ultimately affects women's attitudes and behavior towards others.

## DECISION-MAKING

Success results from decision-making and risk-taking. When we decide what
our most meaningful goals are, success motivates us to accomplish them.

We gain clarity in our lives through making decisions, particularly by establishing priorities. Society provides us with answers. Social norms and expectations guide our decision-making along traditional lines. If we choose to repeat
past patterns, we conform to society's prescriptions. However, if we want to
follow new patterns, we must help to establish new norms and expectations.

New guidelines for women's lives do not appear without being sought. If
women behave unreflectively, they are overwhelmed by powerful influences
culminating in their return to traditional roles. Unless they challenge the norms
of society and decide to do things differently, there can be no modifications or
cultivation of their real interests.

Women must seek new opportunities and options. Awareness must be high
at all times as women define their own realities to challenge the status quo. No
one can do this for them. Only women are sufficiently motivated to assume the
responsibility to free themselves from the restrictions of history and tradition.

The decision to free themselves from traditional roles and life-styles puts
women at risk. Women lose social approval easily when they do things differently or do different things. They risk losing the emotional support and affec-
tion of loved ones by their actions. The knowledge that these are possible and

even predictable consequences of decisions to claim equality requires women to have the courage to pursue their interests.

In other respects, women have nothing to lose from cultivating a habit of more deliberate decision-making. Effective decision-making flows from self-knowledge. Women must know what they want before they can move forward. Self-knowledge empowers women because they interact more satisfactorily with others when they know their strengths and weaknesses.

There are only limited areas of our lives in which we make decisions that have a real impact on ourselves or others. Neither women nor men can influence patterns of interaction without cooperation at some level. Even though it appears that we have little control over our lives, and that social class or gender largely define who we are and the opportunities we have, we always have some freedom to choose how to react or respond to the situations we face.

Women must decide not to succumb to pressures and demands to conform to others' expectations. Unless they deliberately decide and follow through with action, their lives become inextricably entangled with cultural or gender stereotypes.

The most potent areas for women's decisions are identity and commitments. They decide who they are, which commitments they will honor, and how they will honor them. Women's commitments must eventually include active participation in social changes that will free other women to make decisions about their lives. Women cannot merely tell other women that their lives are their total responsibility and let them fend for themselves. They must be available to encourage and support women who want to increase their autonomy and freedom, thereby helping to improve the quality of their lives. They must inevitably decide to help others as well as help themselves through formal and informal intervention, or wide-scale change will be impeded and they will lose their power and strength.

## CHOICES

Decision-making flows from women's options and choices. The way women see their options depends on how they see themselves and the world. Their choices become limited if they think of themselves as weak and ineffective. If they think of themselves as strong or empowered, they are able to define a wide range of options for themselves.

Gains in women's equality result from the choices they think they have. If women identify with power and action rather than with passivity, their choices reflect that decision. Some choices or options for women are listed here.

**1** Success is precluded by allowing ourselves to be fragmented or compartmentalized. A choice to be true to ourselves expresses our real interests more fully than to continuously meet others' needs.

**2** Success depends on individual preferences and choices, and is a planned rather than a chance occurrence. To be successful is to decide what it is that is most important to us, and to act according to these priorities.

**3** Success brings fulfillment and is life-enhancing. We choose success in order to move beyond survival, rather than to receive public acclaim.

**4** Traditional modes of success for women are narrow and restrictive. By choosing to expand their lives, they necessarily carve out new modes of success and new ways of relating to others.

**5** Success changes its meanings through time. We move towards our most important goals in order to experience our most meaningful success.

**6** We choose to be equal, even though our equality may not be recognized. Others may assist us toward success, but our own choice of equal opportunity or equal right to success is crucial.

**7** Women's choice of ideals has a strong influence on their behavior. They modify their behavior by choosing different ideals or values for their identity, commitments, and goals.

**8** New modes of success for women frequently disturb or disrupt others' expectations. Their choice for success predictably generates disapproval. They are inevitably pressured to conform to established ways of doing things, especially by those who are emotionally closest to them.

**9** We must choose success with consideration for others' needs, and in light of what we consider to be our talents and skills. Success is not achievement for one person, but includes giving to others.

**10** Women's choice for success has significant physiological and moral consequences. By not choosing success, they turn away from life rather than live fully and participate in change.

# Chapter 9

# Priorities

It is an accepted limitation of the human condition that we cannot be in all places at the same time, or do all things simultaneously. It is this that necessitates choices and decisions among individuals and within society.

We make our choices with different degrees of awareness. We make thoughtful decisions by considering and deliberating our options according to some standard or preference, or we make automatic, reactive decisions. Valuative acts reinforce our priorities in everyday behavior.

Our priorities may be unique or reflections of the standards of a particular social class or gender. Collective standards are guides for conformity to traditional modes of behavior. To the extent that women's priorities are distinct from men's, women create alternative goals and ways of interacting.

Our priorities sometimes become clearer to us after we make commitments to accomplish certain tasks or participate in specific groups. We gain new views of ourselves and others as we act upon our commitments. Priority assessment is an ongoing activity requiring attention at all times.

Historically, women put others' priorities before or instead of their own. They are late in discovering that they have priorities. They invest tremendous efforts in supporting and assisting others, typically husbands and children, so that those family members may accomplish their own priorities. Although service for loved ones may be a deliberately chosen priority, sacrificing oneself to family and community ultimately generates dissatisfaction or resentment.

Social class or age influence priorities in different ways at various stages of life. Subsistence-level survival absorbs all the priorities of women and men with few economic or energy resources. When material and energy resources are sufficient, it is easier to make constructive contributions to society. Socioeconomic resources and high energy levels increase contributions of ideas as well as material goods.

Our priorities are our most important values. Whenever we self-consciously decide what is most important or meaningful to us, we make value choices. Our dominant priorities or values define our perceptions of ourselves and the world about us, and are strong influences on our behavior. If we value health and well-being, our behavior leads us to achieve these priorities.

Throughout childhood and early adulthood, women are socialized and programmed to accept others' priorities as their own. Maturity and responsibility require, then, that we reassess our priorities as well as establish new priorities. Self-scrutiny is necessary to a full life. If we internalize the priorities of others and fail to cultivate our own, either we find ourselves at the mercy of others' biddings, or we become mere extensions of others. We are fulfilled only when we assume responsibility for choosing and establishing our own priorities.

The process through which women come to know and realize their priorities frequently leads to confrontations and impasses in their negotiations with men. Men predictably resist change as they perceive their status to be threatened by shifts in women's behavior. When women assess and change their priorities, habitual or normative patterns in their exchanges and negotiations with men are upset. Men resist the demise of their privileges, and are thus forced to enter into new negotiations of values with women. When no agreement about priorities is reached, values become nonnegotiable.

Women seek support from other women for the realization of their new priorities. Triadic exchanges between two women and one man illustrate a microcosm of the functions of networks formed by women. Clinical data show that triads or triangles are more stable than dyads, and that relationships between women and men can be supported and strengthened by increased interaction between women.

## STANDARDS

Survival needs force human beings to articulate sets of shared standards based on an understanding of the universe. Religion is one of our most widely accepted resources for imbuing life with meaning. Deities are ascribed with absolute and enduring virtues. Different societies name these absolutes differently—

as God, Truth, Eternal Life, Love, or Justice, for example. Concepts of deities are congruent with particular views of life. Cosmologies define human beings as integral parts of an eternal universe that includes animal, vegetable, and mineral life.

Although people disagree on the specific substance of these supreme values, the concept of absolutes or standards is useful and meaningful. The world and our lives are not products of infinite relative conditions. There is order in the universe which is knowable. Thus one standard or absolute related to our lives is the value we place on life itself. In order to function, we must make assumptions about nature and human nature. These result from our education, wisdom, or enlightment.

Cross-cultural data show immense diversity and versatility in humankind. This range in human essence and responsiveness notwithstanding, there are some common denominators of the human condition that can be a basis for standards. All people need certain conditions to be met in order to survive, and additional conditions to develop their potential. Quality of life can be conceptualized as a continuum between survival and fulfillment—between a life that is endured or one that is enjoyed. If we value the highest quality of human life possible, we can use full development of potential as a standard against which to measure or rate quality of life.

An ideal society would enhance human life by enabling individual members to realize their capacities. It would ensure that every person developed their potential to the fullest. Reference to ideals or standards of this kind allows us to evaluate our options effectively and establish meaningful priorities. Other standards or ideals—such as love, truth, and justice—flow from the assumptions we make about life and human nature.

We understand ourselves more comprehensively through our efforts to understand society and the universe. We become objective about ourselves and our existence only by viewing our lives from the broadest possible perspective. It is from these angles that women know themselves most completely. To some extent women are men and men are women—we are all integral parts of a life and creation which go beyond sex, gender, and interpersonal concerns.

Our standards become a foundation for our lives. This foundation is most viable when our standards incorporate values we choose to honor through our commitments. When we acknowledge what our standards are, we are able to establish our priorities and commitments effectively and define identity clearly. This basic structure of our lives and activity must be considered at all times if we are to be fulfilled.

Standards open our minds to a universe beyond the facts and appearances of our daily lives, giving us stability and security in rapidly changing times. Ultimately our standards define reality for us, and underlie our assumptions and what we take for granted. We prefer one thing or another as a consequence of the standards we choose.

## UNIQUENESS

Every person is unique, having characteristics and special talents which enrich the quality of life in their communities. Our distinctive qualities make us who we are. Identity is a bridging, balancing mechanism incorporating both individuality and universality. We are uniquely ourselves and different from others, and at the same time we belong to the human race. Both aspects of being must be honored through action for the full development of potential.

Women must respect and value their uniqueness in order to maximize their growth and their contributions to society. They have been very powerfully socialized to conform to particular roles and expectations. An integral part of the feminine ethic is to meet, or at least to react to, others' needs and demands. Under these influences women have tended habitually to conform to traditional dictates, especially in their intense efforts to be a "good" woman. The behavior considered by both women and men to be most appropriate for women is female self-sacrifice. This is ultimately a denial and annihilation of women's uniqueness.

Women must deliberately cultivate and strengthen their distinctive qualities to bring balance into their lives. This need is a physiological and a moral imperative. Unless women give serious attention to developing their uniqueness, their behavior will become increasingly restricted, ultimately demonstrating physiological symptoms such as disease or chronic self-destruction.

To neutralize the traditional socialization of women's subordination, a balance of perspectives and action towards uniqueness must be achieved through strategies. Women's choices are neither automatic nor superficial. Women must decide whether to move towards life and expansiveness, or towards restriction, half-living, or death. Neither path will be easy or painless. Counteracting traditional expectations demands considerable emotional resources, energy, and stamina. It is easier for women to continue doing what they and their female ancestors have long done. Such repetitions, however, eventually bring stress-related penalties and little satisfaction.

As women gain a clearer sense of the importance and significance of their uniqueness, they are more able to value, protect, and treasure that central part of themselves. Talents grow and become stronger through deliberate development and broadened applications. Contributions historically confined to domestic milieus are extended to communities and society. When women foster their uniqueness, giving to others becomes more valuable and valued.

Part of women's coming into their own uniqueness is to examine what they really believe and value. By reflecting upon their deepest values, they understand their priorities more fully, and are able to question their desirability and necessity. Women's uniqueness is a guide to this assessment of their standards, and the establishment of identity and commitments. In order to be fully alive, women must know who they really are and must acknowledge their relatedness to all humankind.

## CONTINUITY IN VALUATING

Values are difficult to observe and define through external indicators. Behavior inevitably manifests a person's priorities, and can be thought of as implying an individual's values. Clinical sociologists assess a person's values by gathering information about decisions made and actions taken over long periods of time. The term *value* sums up sociologists' clinical judgments about valuating behavior within the context of a life course.

Value choices continue throughout identity empowerment. To know our present values and future goals requires us to assess our circumstances and decide the extent of change needed. Either our values stay the same for a lifetime, or we decide to change our loyalties. Conflict between our direction in life and that of others may be destructive. Only by scrutinizing our action and interaction can we avoid wasting energies and resources.

We inevitably make value judgments throughout our lives, but we may or may not be aware of the choices we make, or of the consistencies in our decisions. Identity empowerment is a process through which we become aware of our value judgments. This process allows us to realize the different levels at which we make decisions. We approach life by exercising more choices and by making effective decisions about the thoughts, feelings, and actions we want to cultivate and express in our relationships.

Effectiveness in establishing priorities in our lives depends on our skill in checking whether or not we demonstrate consistent standards in our actions. Continuity in valuating is a prerequisite for the establishment of priorities. It is impossible to understand ourselves without continuously making observations and value judgments.

As creatures of habit, we need stable standards by which to assess our circumstances. Whether or not our standards reflect our preferred values, continuity in valuating ensures a consistent awareness and application of standards to different levels of decision-making. Continuity in valuating also heightens our awareness and acknowledgment of our uniqueness. Anything which facilitates knowing who we are at a deep level empowers identity. Deliberate efforts to cultivate the identity we prefer focus on valuating behavior and self-discovery. Most people outside a clinical setting do not observe themselves in action, thereby implicitly deciding to accept and reinforce themselves rather than to change.

Historically women have been pressured to compromise their needs and desires, not having the freedom to develop their potential on their own terms. Valuating is the essence of a necessary continuity in efforts to give birth to self. Women resolve to be who they are, and consequently are less daunted by others' expectations or pressures to conform to traditional models of behavior.

Empowerment is most likely to result from continuity and persistence. Women must persist in their valuating if they are to be successful in creating a meaningful identity for themselves. They must also be prepared for setbacks and resistance to their forward movement. Only when continuity in their valuating neutralizes others' pressures can women be thought of as having confidently established identity in their own right.

## SACRIFICING SELF

Unless women protect themselves with knowledge and deliberate application of their own priorities, they merge with others and lose their uniqueness and distinctiveness. Loss of their priorities, or a lack of awareness of their standards, is tantamount to self-annihilation. Women take change of their lives by establishing and being true to their own priorities. Integrity is acting according to one's priorities, not self-sacrificing for others' needs and demands. Only in this way can women emerge intact from the many complexities of today's world.

Historically women placed a high positive value on self-sacrificing. Selflessness has been and continues to be considered by women and men alike the quintessential feminine virtue. Clinical data demonstrate, however, that women cannot sacrifice self in the long run without sacrificing their own well-being. Unless women have a clearly defined center of identity and commitments in their daily lives, they ultimately experience self-sacrifice as self-destruction.

One means of self-sacrifice has been for women to define themselves in terms of roles rather than as whole human beings. Women and men are more than the sum of the roles they assume. To choose roles freely, rather than blindly to follow roles and their dictates, is vital for a full life.

Women must change the historical pattern of the narrowness and restrictiveness of the few roles that constitute the substance of their lives. Men's roles are more diverse and expansive, with fewer major conflicts or contradictions among their related expectations. Women not only tend to get trapped in the inconsistencies of the roles assigned to them, but they also assume personal responsibility for conflicts intrinsic to those roles. Women's self-esteem is lowered dramatically by the large number of unreasonable demands of traditional role expectations on their resources and energies. Self-sacrificing can be prevented by increasing women's awareness of ways in which they sabotage their efforts to live fully. Friendship and exchanges with other women reduce the probability that they will continue to self-sacrifice. When women cannot discern their own interests clearly, sharing their views with other women enables them to be more objective about their lives.

Any increase in women's detachment from the demands and needs of family members is empowering. This detachment allows them to function autonomously in making decisions about enacting particular roles. Although women friends who give emotional support do not determine the direction in their lives, these friends help them to recognize self-sacrificing and self-destructive behavior.

The processes that culminate in self-sacrifice are debilitating and run counter to empowerment. When women focus on the primary importance of identity and commitments in their lives, these become effective counters to magnifying self-sacrificing tendencies. The solution to women's negative programming is to establish life-affirming priorities clearly and decisively.

The more women articulate their own standards for judgments about life, and the more they honor their uniqueness, the more likely they are to let go of their participation in destructive patterns of interaction, such as self-sacrificing. Women must continue to assess their priorities and make conscious decisions about their values in identity if they are to recover from past patterns of self-sacrificing. Only in this way can they turn their lives around.

## DEVELOPING POTENTIAL

The goal of developing potential is achieved by decisive efforts to make the most of ourselves in any given circumstances. For example, we may choose education as a means of developing potential. This is essentially a drawing forth of our talents and capabilities. However, developing potential is more than an intellectual or intraphysic process. We need to interact with others in order to be more of what we are or in order to change ourselves.

Women have historically assumed the responsibility to nurture others, and more specifically, to motivate their children to be upwardly mobile. Only recently have women cared enough about themselves to nurture each other, and to encourage each other to develop their potential. Women can be themselves most effectively when they have purpose, direction, or goals in their lives. It is this movement forward that pulls them out of their narrow, restrictive sense of self, and allows them to bridge their uniqueness and their universal characteristics.

Women's priorities set the scene for the most effective ways to develop their potential. When they know which of their values are most important to them, they define a foundation for their identity and a frame of reference for their development of potential. Making the most of their skills and talents gives women power, and having a clear sense of identity makes their use of this power effective.

Education may change women's values imperceptibly, significantly, or dramatically. By acquiring knowledge they put their lives in a broader perspective and are able to see themselves and their world differently. Education reduces women's parochialism and ethnocentrism. Although education may broaden their perspectives so much that all values and structures appear to be relative, in time this dislodging of previous cultural knowledge and wisdom provides the makings for new knowledge and different but stable frames of reference. Women's standards change in this process of adjustment and new standards emerge to guide them in formulating new priorities.

Although each person has her or his own specific goals, the development of potential must be universally valued if we are to improve the quality of life for all. This goal may or may not be deliberately chosen, but it is important at some level for many human beings. Expressing our strengths is a vital aspect of living fully and doing so enhances life satisfaction.

Women's development of potential creates cooperative patterns of behavior which contrast with competitive modes established by men. Women help each other strengthen their capabilities. They know that they are less likely to make progress in developing their potential if they do so at the expense of others, as men have done in the past. By extending nurturing skills to each other, women establish new patterns of interaction in communities and society.

Women's need to develop potential is imperative, not superfluous. They develop potential in order to gain or maintain equality and to live satisfactorily. Developing potential moves women into life. If they do not develop potential, their lack of active responsiveness to the status quo results in their continuing engulfment in patriarchal values and structures. Identity empowerment is effective in arresting or reversing these annihilating processes because it motivates women to participate in society equally and on their own terms.

## CLASS AND MOBILITY

Women's life-chances vary according to their social class. In short, women who belong to lower social classes generally have more limited life-chances than women who belong to higher social classes. It is largely economic resources that either confine lower-class women's activities or increase possibilities for women in higher social classes. Although women's life-styles are extremely varied, there are certain dependency consistencies. Women who are economically independent and self-supporting have more expansive lives than women who are economically dependent.

It is crucial for women to have their own means of support, regardless of social-class standing. Independent economic resources, whether earned or inherited, allow women autonomy in their decision-making and activities. Where women, including those in the upper class, are economically dependent on men, their lives can be totally disrupted by a man's decision to withhold resources.

Women's emotional independence from men flows from and is sustained by economic independence. As women become economically independent, they become more emotionally independent. Whatever their social class, economic independence is a prerequisite for women's identity empowerment and the development of their potential.

Women in upper classes are frequently more economically dependent on men than women in lower classes. Married women in these status groups grow accustomed to their husbands' high salaries, and simultaneously tend to devalue their skills to carve out a profession, occupation, or societal contribution of their own. The imbalance in economic assets between spouses in the upper class results in emotional imbalance in the couple's relationship. The person with the higher income generally dominates decisions and the establishment of family priorities.

Middle-class women are more likely to have been motivated to pursue a career for themselves than upper-class women. Although this may present conflicts for middle-class women in other areas of their lives, clinical and family research data indicate that consistent economic rewards from work outside the home sustain their emotional independence in intimate relationships. While professional women are no less needy for love and attention than are other women, they are generally less vulnerable to male domination.

Lower-class women continuously struggle for survival. Sociological research has documented that lower-class women frequently work harder than lower-class men, especially in minority groups. These women may be economically independent, but their very limited economic resources make them emotionally unequal and vulnerable in their relationships with men in other social classes. Although assets do not have to be precisely equal in order to establish autonomy in personal relationships, sufficient assets should be held by each to allow for upward mobility. This mobility may not be possible for lower-class women.

Identity transcends class lines and can motivate behavior and productivity towards upward mobility. Though not necessarily setting class mobility as a goal, establishing clear goal priorities enables women to seize opportunities for self-expression and achievement. Direction and purpose emerge from these priorities, giving an accelerated and enthusiastic tone to activities no longer dictated by particular class styles.

By seeing and feeling themselves as equal, women transcend patriarchal gender classes. They are a gender class of their own, with socialized distinctions from men. As a class, however, women can be mobile rather than perpetually subordinate to men. Society will not necessarily move towards a matriarchal class system, but traditional patriarchal authority structures and controls will be loosened.

## GENERALIZATIONS AND PROPOSITIONS

Generalizations about priorities in women's identity and commitments follow. These generalizations highlight the importance of establishing priorities for the empowerment of women.

1   Women's real priorities or preferences become standards by which they can assess situations more objectively.

**2** Women develop potential through establishing priorities that give purpose and direction.

**3** Women must continuously assess their priorities and standards as they move forward. The only endpoint to the necessity for scrutinizing valuating behavior for living fully is death.

**4** One priority is for women to see themselves as both members of the human race and unique individuals.

**5** Women must take themselves seriously so as to consolidate their energies and not dissipate resources by sacrificing for others as a lifelong value and commitment.

**6** Economic class membership influences the quality of all women's lives. Economic independence is the most necessary component of women's empowerment.

**7** Gender defines class, but identity promotes mobility beyond the subordination of women.

Specific relationships between individuals and social influences lead towards more effective action for women. These propositions relate to priorities.

**1** Women become more aware of their identity through deliberately selecting their most meaningful priorities.

**2** Cultivating uniqueness leads towards self-empowerment when it is placed within the context of shared participation in the human condition.

**3** We cannot know ourselves without careful observation and scrutiny. Increased self-knowledge increases power and effectiveness in interpersonal or social exchanges.

**4** The less women self-sacrifice, the more they are able to claim their own identity and real interests.

**5** Identity empowerment effectively supplants self-annihilation through excessive personal sacrifice for others' needs.

**6** Development of potential results from identity empowerment.

**7** Priorities allow women to transcend class lines and move effectively towards economic and emotional independence.

# Chapter 10

# Negotiating as an Equal

Women need equal opportunities to lead full lives. Opening up opportunities and possibilities to women does not inevitably take away men's privileges, however. Competition, warfare, and survival of the fittest do not need to prevail. We can create more workable ways of relating to each other in order to be equals.

Equality does not occur without interaction. Women cannot become equal in a vacuum. As values permeate their activities, exchanges with others allow women to know and experience their most important values. Crises, conflicts, or confrontations heighten their awareness of who they are, and increased intensity in interaction causes their deepest values to surface. Our identity determines whether or not we believe ourselves to be equal to those around us. Our expectations of life derive from how we see ourselves and others. When we see each other as equals, we negotiate as equals.

Women change the ways they relate to men when they realize they have as many talents. Understanding the limiting consequences of their gender socialization and programming exposes their false beliefs and frees women. We contribute more of our skills and gifts to others when we conduct ourselves as equals.

Although aspects of equality may be legislated, only when women believe they are equal can they act fully as equals. Education brings about a freer definition of self, and identity choices empower self. When women's awareness is heightened, they are more likely to behave as equals than to perpetuate their subordination. This quality of being allows women to consider how they might most effectively contribute to society.

Although women know themselves to be equals, men do not necessarily change their perceptions of women's subordination. When women interact with men as equals, they tend to be pressured to return to being subordinates. Unless women assert their equality, they revert to habitual patterns in reaction to this pressure.

Women's articulation of goals supports their efforts to achieve equality. By accomplishing social objectives, women demonstrate their talents to society and serve as role models for other women. They do not have to prove themselves through achievement in order to be equal. It is less the accomplishment of women's goals that is important, than their effort and involvement in working toward the goals.

Thus lack of fulfillment and dissatisfaction abate when women move into more equal negotiations. Women empower themselves by identifying with values of their choice and by negotiating these values on an equal basis.

Negotiations pass through many different stages and some negotiations are more intense or more significant than others. Only if equality is practiced consistently are negotiations effective. Equality generates a respect for freedom, and this needs to be maintained at all times and in all circumstances if women are to come into their own. To live fully they must identify with the value of equality and claim equality at deep inner levels of their being.

## EQUAL OPPORTUNITY

The most urgent, viable goal for all women and men is equal opportunity. Equity in all things is impossible given the rich variation of human life and society. Equal access to creative and productive life conditions is attainable though, at least in principle.

Equal opportunity is difficult to define. People have varied material assets and vastly different abilities and capacities. Equal opportunity necessitates a leveling of some kind so that each person begins with the same advantages. Our diversity and contrasts suggest that equal opportunities may have to be earned or legislated in order to be brought into being. Our responsibility is to translate these ideals into action. When women are not strong enough to help themselves to be equal, legal changes can structure increased or enlarged opportunities for them.

Thus external measures, such as more advantageous laws or increased economic resources, may be essential for bringing about real changes for women, especially poor and disadvantaged women. Advantages from creating these kinds of supports and structures occur when women want these changes, and strengthen their views of their own potential sufficiently to benefit from the legislated freedom. Women's status cannot be enhanced unless they are active and willing participants in these processes. In the best of all worlds, their outer and inner lives are synchronized so that they respond actively to opportunities with equal consideration of others.

Clinical data suggest that it is in women's best interest to cultivate attitudes and postures which will enable them to define and promote equal opportunities. Women's beliefs in equality need to become sufficiently sacred to them that they no longer doubt their own worth. This belief allows women to proceed as if they are equals even though factually this may not be accurate. When they are motivated by a clear sense of equality and self-worth, they are more likely to seize opportunities and thrive from them.

Women strengthen their capacity to negotiate effectively as equals when they know that they have availed themselves of opportunities as equals. Equal opportunities flow from women's deep acceptance of their equality rather than from their focusing on injustices in their lives. Inequalities can be found when sought, especially when they are looked for with determination. However, constructive opportunities can also be defined in any situation, whatever the conditions may be. It is by having faith in their equal rights and equal opportunities that women move forward with their lives and make effective progress. If women spend their energy primarily in describing and focusing on the injustices of their lives, they will stay enmeshed in problematic conditions without being able to harness the energies necessary to surface from these limitations and live satisfactorily.

The opposite of opportunity is restriction. Restrictions in women's lives are increasingly well-documented. By definition, restrictions do not allow us to be equal. It is women's challenge and responsibility to transform their restrictions into opportunities for the expression of their innate equality and spirit.

## EQUAL RESOURCES

Equality in resources is not as significant for the development of opportunities as equality in access to resources. We cannot stabilize the distributions of resources sufficiently so that shares remain equal indefinitely. Where structures allow resources to be allocated for specific needs, however, unnecessary inequalities can be avoided or neutralized.

Beliefs in the importance of resources generally emphasize material goods. Another vital resource, especially for women, is ideas and ideals that transcend material inadequacies and limitations. Negative conditioning, such as belief in male supremacy, has prevented women from having equal access to values of strength and power. By examining and deliberately constructing identity, women avail themselves of more active ideals, inspiring them to move forward with their lives.

A primary resource for both women and men is their own ability. Women cope with an alarming range of hazardous life conditions. They continuously establish their equal competence to men, but they are rarely aware of their accomplishment. Women's closeness to procreation through their distinctive bodily functions is also a strength and resource which they tend to overlook.

When women create or strengthen their identity, they increase their resourcefulness. By becoming whole persons they establish their equality with others, being able to act with more confidence than they did previously. Women's resources evolve from their awareness. Their most vital, equalizing resource is their awareness of their own worth.

Women who claim equal access to resources experience well-being rather than restriction. They can be more productive in their lives when they have a secure starting point. When they believe that they are able to handle any situation that might arise, they establish their equal claims to resources and simultaneously move towards a more satisfying life.

Resourceful attitudes may not correlate with external reality, but they motivate us to achieve our ideal goals. Women's perception of the availability of resources strengthens their capacity to aim for the most they can imagine. Knowing they have equal access to resources launches them into making their greatest contributions to others. Indeed, only when women are convinced that they can achieve something will they set out to do it.

Women multiply their resources by pursuing education. When women are intellectually disciplined and well-informed, they organize their resources more effectively. Education links women to the knowledge that underlies their values and culture. Education also informs women about the vast resources that lie beyond their immediate grasp. They broaden their understanding of the world and expand their horizons. They are lifted up beyond the limitations of their immediate domestic and community milieus.

Education is women's means of entry to society, their connection to higher ideals and greater hopes. They have to believe in the resources of education, however, before these resources can be actualized. Satisfaction results from women's ability to use their inner and outer resources. When they believe that no one has the power to separate them from their right of equal access to resources, they are better able to approach them. These expectations mobilize women and the resources they need.

## VALUE OF EQUITY

Women negotiate more effectively as equals if they place a high value on equity. It is not necessary for those with whom they negotiate to value equity also, although consensus creates more open and honest transactions. Women define their own identities and have no power over the identities of others. When they place a high value on equity, they order all their values in relation to equity.

Equity implies inclusiveness. As it is applied to all, it suggests variety and richness within oneness. A balanced pluralism with tolerance and cooperation is the product of interaction among equals. Further, valuing equity promotes a vision of our own and others' wholeness; we feel more complete and can reflect on our lives, society, and the universe. The probability that our activities are integrated, coordinated, and harmonious increases when we place a greater value on equity. Our remaining values are subordinated to the greater value of equity. Fragmentation, compartmentalization, and complementarity are neutralized or dissolved by emphases on wholeness and equity.

Equity is thus a constructive, life-enhancing goal. By consistently moving towards equity, and acting as equals, we grow to greater maturity. Because women have been programmed to be subordinate to men, it takes self-conscious effort to move into equality, otherwise when they act automatically, they function as subordinates rather than as equals. It is only when equity is applied in action that equality is expressed effectively.

Valuing equity makes many things possible. When we believe ourselves to be as worthwhile as all others, we are motivated to achieve a wide range of objectives. A belief in equity allows us to be led more by inner promptings than by external pressures, and values enable us to transcend roles and structures in our lives. Equity eases or even neutralizes limitations. Women's shift in attention and values creates dramatic changes in their lives as they are transformed from victims of circumstances to actors in modifying restrictive roles and social structures.

Our inner resources improve our functioning and relationships with others. Clinical data suggest that the influence of spiritual strength outweighs the influence of physical strength in our lives, and that spiritual strength is magnified by placing a value on equity. We express and strengthen the value we place on equity by negotiating with others as equals. We cannot be equal to others unless we interact as equals. Equality results from action rather than from thinking and analysis.

The value of equity becomes an ideal which has practical consequences for daily behavior. We deal with crises more confidently when we place a high positive value on equity. We transcend pain and turmoil when we deliberately incorporate a value of equity in our behavior and commitments. A conscious cultivation of the value of equity moves us beyond narrow definitions of self. We become more at one with the universe when we live out our sense of equity as a primary value. Equity becomes a foundation for identity which cannot be substantially shaken by tumultuousness in everyday life. We can safely base our activities and commitments on this value, as equity underlies diversity in humankind. The value of equity can be trusted as an organizing principle for our lives.

## PRIVILEGES AND RESOURCES

Privilege is based on unequal resource distribution. Women are born into inequalities of privileges and resources that characterize their lives until they die. Privileges and resources mark the external, objective aspects of our reality and ourselves. It is essentially in our inner, subjective lives that we know our equality and negotiate with others as equals. Through this knowledge we tap into our deepest levels of verbal and nonverbal communication, and express ourselves with the utmost honesty and openness.

Negotiating as an equal requires that we see ourselves as important as those who dominate us, and as unimportant as those who are less privileged or poorer than we are. Negotiating as an equal requires that we see beyond the facts of external appearances and know a level of reality where each person has equal worth. In this state of being we acknowledge others for who they are and allow them to be themselves. Respect and tolerance for others increases as we accept their equal right to live a satisfying life.

We cannot make judgments about who people are by assessing only their external, objective privileges and resources. Those with high social status, advanced education, and economic assets wield considerable power and influence over others. They will not, however, be able to sustain others' respect unless they allow or even encourage others to be themselves.

Traditionally men have been evaluated according to external indicators of privilege and resources, with less attention to their accompanying responsibilities. As most women have historically lived without substantial privileges and resources, their attention has habitually focused more on the inner dimensions of character. Women spend so much time and energy respecting others, however, that they pay insufficient attention to building self-respect. Focus on others decreases their equality and self-worth, devalues their contributions to others, and obfuscates their own particular privileges and resources.

By consciously cultivating identity, women neutralize this tendency to deny their self-worth. Assessing skills and talents, and placing a value on their own privileges and resources, makes women more likely to enter into negotiations as equals. Identity empowerment is a process whereby women define their own privileges and resources, standing by them in all negotiations.

In order to define identity adequately, women select values they are prepared to uphold whatever the circumstances. In this way a few of their values become nonnegotiable, and they may express their allegiance to them more fully and intensely than survival needs. Living fully flows from purposeful living and cannot occur if women are inattentive to their own privileges and resources in their equal relations with others.

Women redefine privileges and resources to include inner dimensions of their lives. Although they still need social assurances of status, it is their inner strengths that enable them to move toward more visible social participation.

Privileges and resources are multifaceted and they enrich the lives of all at different levels of reality and communication.

## COOPERATION OR COMPETITION

Modern feminist values espouse a new model of social process. Women strengthen their capacity to cooperate with each other through support networks. Although women in patriarchal societies consistently compete with each other for limited material privileges and resources, they must counter this conditioning to attain increased fulfillment and satisfaction. Women's relationships with each other are a primary source of cooperative negotiations. Instead of pursuing the same goals as other women, they carve out their own. This process allows them to express their own values and talents directly as well as to contribute to community and society. In this cooperation women negotiate as equals, strengthening themselves and their contributions to others.

A less developed stage of change, but one in which women are also pioneers, is the establishment of more cooperative relationships with men. When women accept patriarchal values, they participate in more destructive modes of competition with women and men. When they negotiate as equals with men, they initiate cooperative modes of negotiations and increase the possibility of satisfaction for both women and men.

Cooperation includes nurturing, support, and mutual respect. By contrast, competition is a deliberate disregard of others to attain a disproportionate share of privileges and resources. A negative consequence of competition is that all cannot have benefits and some receive inadequate shares.

Competition is a power phenomenon. We are trained to pursue the same goals as others, and power is given to those who achieve the most, regardless of others' needs. Competition is rationalized as necessary for survival; we think of the fittest as being those who survive the rigors of competition.

A major disadvantage of competition is that we view one another with hostility. We are not able to work effectively with our competitors so we pursue the same goals as others in divisive ways. Hostility is perpetuated by competition, as expressed by aggression, resentment, alienation, and isolation. When we are not equipped to compete, we tend to give up or drop out. Sociological research postulates that apathy and passivity are increased in competitive mass societies.

Cooperation has distinct advantages. Not characterized by competitive negotiations between unequals, cooperation approximates the ideal of negotiations between equals. In contrast to competitive negotiations, cooperative relations are not centered around self-interest and individual achievement. Rather, they are reciprocal exchanges among equals with the clearly defined intentions of contributing to each other through meeting community and societal needs.

This portrayal of women's cooperative negotiations is idealistic. It illustrates feminist principles in action in favorable conditions. We must have some vision of possibilities, however, in order to bring about significant change or improvement in the quality of life for larger numbers of people. Cooperation would reduce the isolation and alienation of women and men alike. As they cannot mutually coexist, we must move away from competition in order to move toward cooperation.

## CONSEQUENCES OF NEGOTIATING AS AN EQUAL

There are individual and social consequences of negotiating as an equal. Women strengthen their operating positions by holding their own as equals in their household and family milieus. Conditioning makes women believe themselves unequal, even within the context of their own homes and families. Their decisions to interact as equals allows women to get beyond this subordination. An eventual consequence of negotiating as an equal within a family is the stabilization and balancing of key relationships. A societal consequence of negotiating as an equal is improvement in women's status.

Identity is empowered by continuously negotiating as an equal. Equality is eventually gained by assuming our equal rights in attitude if not in action. Feeling ourselves to be equal eventually motivates us to take action as an equal.

We clarify our values through negotiations. We modify and strengthen our values and commitments as we interact. Our intellectual analysis of who we are is animated when we know what it is we stand for, and how far we will go to meet others' expectations and demands. Our underlying belief in our own equality influences our patterns of interaction. When there is a marked discrepancy between women's habitual subordination and their new equality, dramatic shifts in their behavior must follow. Under such circumstances, there is bound to be even greater resistance and reaction to women's new equality. The more dramatic the change they make in claiming equality, the more pressure they will have to deal with in maintaining this posture.

Negotiating as an equal transforms our value systems and sense of identity. By defining and following new opportunities to be equal, women improve their access to established resources and create new kinds of privileges and resources for themselves. They move from being victims of circumstance to being able to transcend some of the restrictions and inequalities of past conditions and programming. Negotiating as an equal results, then, in a gradual transformation of structures of competition, replacing them with cooperative modes of interacting.

Negotiating as equals implies tolerance and respect for others. Authoritarian structures are loosened and life moves with a flow of reciprocity in conditions of equal negotiations. Social structures and processes become "organic" or flexible when we negotiate as equals.

Some of the formal changes that occur from negotiating as equals include realistic and balanced legislation as well as reflective ways of dealing with major world problems such as peace and development. Nurturing feminine values heightens social awareness, and social processes become more balanced. Women move closer to other women, and women and men are more able to work meaningfully in partnership ventures and in other kinds of cooperative teamwork.

Negotiating as an equal has specific empirical consequences. Clinical family data show that these consequences depend upon the context and longevity of identity modification. While these repercussions differ, it is clear that more people could ultimately benefit from negotiations between equals, particularly in the context of family interaction. Negotiations between equals enhance life and move us out of dangerously imbalanced relationships and structures.

## GENERALIZATIONS AND PROPOSITIONS

Generalizations about negotiating as an equal are necessarily tentative as widespread conditions of equality do not yet exist. Clinical data define results of micro level shifts in women's status from subordination to equality. Social trend data more directly related to feminist movements illustrate ways in which broader scale changes occur.

1   We define more opportunities for ourselves by resolving to negotiate as equals with others.

2   Negotiating as equals diminishes institutionalized inequalities.

3   Negotiating as equals is a basic value in identity which promotes a reordering of other values.

4   Negotiating as an equal strengthens access to resources and redefines our understanding and acceptance of privilege.

5   Negotiating as equals gradually transforms competition to cooperation.

6   Women promote legislation for equality indirectly by being equal in everyday situations.

7   We promote more solutions to world problems by acting as equals. Interpersonal behavior has historical consequences which go beyond personal milieus.

Propositions suggest ways in which negotiations as equals can be accomplished and the nature of their consequences. Processes and outcomes indicate the following relationships between influences.

1   A major outcome of identity empowerment is more consistent and effective negotiation as an equal with all others.

2   Identity is further empowered as we negotiate as equals. Identity must be empowered through action.

**3** When we negotiate as equals, we enter into more satisfying commitments. Only satisfying commitments endure through time, and continuity enhances the meaning of our lives.

**4** To the extent that negotiations among women and between women and men become more equal, competitive social structures are replaced by cooperative social structures.

**5** In order to negotiate effectively as an equal, our relationships must be based on equity and a belief in our own equality. This priority or value choice necessitates a reordering of all our values and a reorganization of social values.

**6** New resources and privileges flow from our active claims to more equal statuses. When we change our power and influence in relationships and in society, we redefine established modes of success.

**7** Negotiating as an equal is a fundamental principle in micro and macro social processes, with the potential to change attitudes, values, and social structures.

# Chapter 11

# Friendship

Families are a major source of companionship and enjoyment in modern society. However, as cities become ever more impersonal, nonfamily friendships become more essential. Indeed, both women and men increasingly need friends in order to be secure and fulfilled.

It becomes easier to assess who our friends are when we clarify our identity. We may keep friends for a lifetime as well as make new friends in changing circumstances. Whatever the motivation or purpose for cultivating friendships, clinical data show that we strengthen self by having a circle of at least six friends. Our friendship networks give us intimacy, meaning, and emotional sustenance.

Women have particular needs and styles of friendship. Friendships among women are very important because these exchanges deepen their understanding of the influence of expectations and conflicts in their lives. Friendships also promote possibilities for increasing their strength and mutual support. Women are encouraged and inspired when they develop identity through expressing their real interests.

Women also need friendships with men. Men are not the enemy, and many benefits accrue from relating to men as brothers, as well as through the more traditional roles of lover and spouse. It is only when women and men know how to deal with each other honestly, cooperatively, and creatively that their best and strongest identities will be realized.

Ideas, thoughts, and feelings are important substantive exchanges in friendships. We choose our friends more meaningfully when we make deliberate value choices for identity since our preferences flow from our sense of self. Further, we see ourselves more clearly through our friends' perspectives. In short, our friends reflect us or complement us.

Family research shows that because we choose our friends, it is easier to love them than to love family members. However, friendships are intrinsically more brittle than families. The best of friends are much more likely to disappear overnight for no apparent reason than are relatives. We must work on our friendships to keep and strengthen them. Much has to be discussed and lived through if friends are to be counted on.

Nurturing and caring for others characterize women's roles and values. Women have long excelled in nurturing and in placing this caring above other activities. Clinical research shows that because they give of themselves more fully, women sustain better friendships than do men. There is not doubt that women can use their skills and experience in nurturing to their advantage. They can choose friends who have their interests at heart rather than those who are overly dependent on them and exploit their concern. Women are recharged through constructive friendships and depleted by unnecessary dependencies.

It is essential to have friends in a mobile, impersonal society. Whether our mobility is geographical, educational, professional, or all three, our innate interdependence requires that we look to others for strength. Women's isolation and loneliness, experienced particularly in suburban life-styles, have precipitated a wide variety of personal and social ills, ranging from depression to destructive behavior. Friendship helps us to break out of uncomfortable and unhealthy circumstances, and leads towards developing our potential and enriching our lives.

## FAMILY OR FRIENDS?

Gender role researchers view the family as a major site of oppression for women. Women are socialized to place primary emphasis on the family and to respect and honor as supreme the specific family roles assigned to them. Before the 19th century, many men worked at home, and by virtue of their presence participated in parenting and some domestic decision-making. Since the industrial revolution, when men moved their work away from the home, women have been expected to serve most of the needs and demands of family members.

In times of modernization women continue to be committed to domestic milieus. When they define their obligations solely in terms of the family, women devote an inordinate amount of time and energy to these tasks, building a mental and emotional boundary between family activities and the outside world. Women's commitments to family responsibilities remain, whether women actually spend most of their time at home or work away from their families.

Women's liberation must therefore occur within the family as well as in society. Liberation does not require women to ignore family needs, or deliberately avoid marriage and parenthood, as these are viable options. Liberation gives women autonomy, and they can claim this freedom in the midst of family life. Identity clarification moves women towards liberation and away from burdensome family demands.

While women's emotional resources are most severely stressed within their families, paradoxically, they are also most able to carve out meaningful and lasting freedom for themselves within their domestic milieu. Household chores suppress women's creativity, but at the same time clinical data confirm that women's interaction with family members promotes more dramatic shifts in their identity than their interaction with people at work. Women's parents and their parents' families remain a significant influence on their lives. By contrast, when women's husbands and children are unable to withstand the impact of women's different patterns of behavior, these families may disintegrate.

To the extent that women effectively endure pressures and stresses, they free themselves from the demands of their families. Autonomy in relation to their families enables them to claim their freedom more easily in other social settings.

Friendship, particularly friendship with other women, is a bridge for women to use in distancing themselves from their overinvolvement with family concerns. Meaningful connections outside the immediate family increase women's understanding and support in their quest for fuller living. The additional resource of friendship enhances women's self-respect, and leads towards their discovery of increased options for identity beyond the traditional roles of daughter, wife, and mother. Although it is essential for women to interact with their parents, sisters, and brothers to be fully aware of themselves, friends are an invaluable source for clarifying identity and commitments.

Still, the essential process of changing perceptions and behavior by expressing values in action is more effective when it occurs in the context of women's families than in the context of their friends. Family members continue to interact with each other through different generations, and their dependence ensures that they will not cut off all communication.

Unlike our relatives, our friends have no continuing obligations or ties to each other. Only in extraordinary circumstances does friendship continue under stress. We are blessed by our families, not because they love us or we love them, but because they are there. We might run away or be disowned, but in most cases they remain a significant reference group and our deepest source of emotional dependence.

## IDENTIFICATION THROUGH FRIENDS

Self-discovery results from observing, reflecting, and acting rather than solely from thinking. We need to become more objective about ourselves in order to see our options and make choices. This is difficult given our subjectivity and the pervasiveness of values. Values are personal, interpersonal,and universal. We define ourselves and the world about us through our value choices, and our selection of friends results from these choices. What we find attractive about others is expressed overtly or covertly in our own lives. We make friends with people or with those who seem to be who we want to be.

We define who we are through our friendships. We may find that our expectations are not being met in the course of our friendships—our friends may reflect our weaknesses rather than our strengths. This situation frequently ends friendships. Deciding not to be a friend is a significant way to understand ourselves. We identify ourselves more clearly when we adhere to our most important values in our friendships.

Friends are particularly helpful to women who are committed to heightening their awareness of self. Self-revelation occurs through the many conversations and nonverbal interactions over long periods of time. These exchanges touch deep levels of self that might not otherwise be experienced. Our innermost beliefs, thoughts, and feelings are articulated when friends make time to listen to us.

Identity is clarified for each woman when experiences are shared, especially when there are parallels in their lives. Differences between friends also contribute towards clarifying identity and defining how our lives and values contrast with theirs.

Self-discovery and the empowerment of self are more likely to occur in times of crisis than during the course of everyday activity. We are fortunate if we can turn to friends for strength and support when our lives are disrupted. One danger is that friendships become overburdened by intense needs, especially in crises. To the extent that friends help to sustain us when our deepest convictions are shaken, their unique views and assurances are vital for transcending crises and gaining self-knowledge.

Patterns of exchanges with friends depend on external circumstances. We may meet friends in person, talk to them by telephone, write to them, or stay with them from time to time. Whatever the structures we create for these communications, we benefit from friendships most by maintaining an awareness of our own deep internal transformations. Priorities are clarified as friends respond to reports of our experiences and perceptions.

We associate friends with particular stages of our lives although we may have lifetime friends. When we change our behavior, however, it is difficult to sustain the same degree of meaningful exchange with our friends. We must constantly be ready to renew friendship—with the same friends or new friends. Although we are saddened to let go of old friends, moving forward in life is more important. Our needs and values change as we empower self, and we are attracted to different kinds of people at different stages of our lives. If we want to live as fully as possible, we should not try to hold on to our friends or allow ourselves to be held back by them.

We always care about our friends, particularly those who stand by us in major crises, so friendship can be renewed at any time. We give rebirth to each other through friendship, and embrace the fresh and new in our lives through strengths gained.

## CHANGING FRIENDS

To some extent our friends change in spite of us rather than because of us. If we are upwardly mobile, we make new contacts and acquaintances who become closer to us than earlier friends. We may choose to keep our old friends, making persistent efforts to maintain those friendships whatever the circumstances.

We do not usually end friendship without sound reasons. However, women need to be objective about their friendships so they can assess their worth. They must be active participants in their friendships without being overly adaptive. The perpetuation of friendships that debilitate rather than enhance one's energies erodes identity and destroys self. Self-respect must be preserved or cultivated through our selection of friends and friendship styles. We need to get on with our lives and live more fully through our friends, consciously avoiding negative friendship patterns.

When we look at our personal histories, we appreciate the attention given by friends at particular times. If we are able to maintain meaningful contact with these people, self-enrichment results. In return, we like to be available to them, especially in times of need. We may not strive to maintain such friendships at all times, however, or try to resolve relationship problems in the course of the friendship because this is not the primary reason we associate with this friend.

We can neither afford to become estranged from our friends nor to pursue them. When our friendships are not mutually supportive or enriching and strengthening, it is more likely that they will not endure. Given the fact that healthy needs for companionship are met by reciprocity, continuity of friendship depends to a large extent on equal participation and full partnership.

Friendship is an important guide for women seeking equality. We reach for egalitarian ideals in our closest friendships by working through dependency concerns. If this is not possible, we may have to change friends. We decide to stay in friendships or move away to make new friends depending on how we identify ourselves and on how much we value self.

We cannot change other people, we can only change ourselves. If our best efforts to give of ourselves in friendship do not work, we have a responsibility to find new friends who will meet our needs for companionship. We must let go of friendships that do not move towards equality, refusing to manipulate or coerce others to do as we would want. We need to give each friend as much respect and freedom as possible, as these are essential for equality. Our only choice may be to let go of those friends who do not give us basic respect and freedom.

The loss of friends, even by choice, is generally painful. Our need for friends is based on many human needs. When we cling to old values and identities, we also cling to old friends who embody our original preferences and life-styles. As we loosen old ties, we become freer and more liberated. New friends are found and they respond to deeper levels of our awareness and being. We move forward knowing that our companionship needs will be met.

## NURTURING VALUES

Women are conditioned to love and care for others through their traditional responsibilities as wife and mother. As daughters, women are expected to look after aging relatives, particularly parents. These values of loving and caring are so deep-seated, however, that they dissipate energies that could be focused on women's own lives.

Women decrease the probability of becoming a victim of burdensome care-taking responsibilities by pulling away from family demands through friendship. Giving attention to one's needs for friends has a balancing effect on family responsibilities. Ideally, the friends women choose will nurture them. Women, as well as other members of their families, need to grow and become stronger.

Nurturing values motivate women to be responsive whatever the circumstances. They protect those they love until they are able to protect themselves. In carrying out their many different kinds of responsibilities, however, women need to have friends they can count on.

Women's empathy and deep mutual understanding for each other lead to caring friendships. When women lead increasingly expansive lives, they identify with groups other than the family and with values other than those which reflect their former loyalties. Women's mobility results from stretching their contacts to all parts of society. Nurturing values are expressed through interaction with women they do not know, as well as with those who are emotionally close. This pattern broadens women's base of security and empowers them.

Traditionally nurturing family members is the center of women's morality. Making friends is an alternative to the expression of these values. The scope of women's friendships presents an almost infinite variety of possibilities. Each time a woman makes a friend, she creates a new direction for her life.

The deliberate expression of nurturing values through friendships allows women to bridge private and public spheres of interaction. Historically women were banished to private domains, not having rights to participate in public arenas. Expressing nurturing values in friendship increases women's security. They reduce their estrangement and competition with other women by expressing more positive forms of dependency. Clinical data suggest that sufficiently pervasive egalitarian friendships can decrease existing antagonisms among individuals and within societies.

Women must also direct their attention to self-development. They can nurture or be nurtured, but in the final analysis they must be capable and willing to tend to their own needs. This creative regeneration of personal resources is not self-indulgent; self-knowledge accompanies attentiveness to oneself. We can only love others fully when we look after ourselves.

A feminist belief is that women's strengths in expressing nurturing values contribute toward saving our world from destruction. This impact can only be achieved by consolidating women's resources because we have reached the limits of utilizing male values effectively. Women's nurturing values redress the imbalances of current social priorities and resource allocations. In order to move onward, social values must be more inclusive, incorporating nurturing values in exchanges far beyond the family.

## WORKING ON FRIENDSHIP

Women thrive more from friendships that express vested interest in their well-being than from friendships that require self-sacrifice or an overextension of self. Well-being is ultimately derived from personal growth and strengthening self. Identity clarification may become one of many motivating factors in choosing and making friends.

Growth within friendships is not easily attained. Each person has strong dependency cravings as well as a need for self-expression, and both must be honored to define identity. However, the expression of our differences may lead to conflict.

Working on friendship thus means acknowledging the similarities and differences between ourselves and our friends. Paradoxically, by recognizing the importance of our mutual distinctiveness, we become closer to others. Friendships are more rewarding and more supportive when we maintain some focus on self rather than allow ourselves to be sidetracked or diverted by friends' needs.

It is necessary to have sufficient self-awareness at all times to be consistent in our interactions with friends. We cultivate identity successfully when we no longer constantly change our allegiances or characteristic ways of behaving. We shape identity according to our deepest values, and it is only shifts in those values that bring about changes in identity. We no longer change to placate others, including our friends.

Women's focus on identity predictably precipitates conflict in some friendships. Where there is insufficient breathing space in friends' sharing, or lack of depth of understanding, the friendship will be brittle. In some cases friendships may be so precarious that they cannot withstand conflict or they disintegrate after short periods of conflict. Friendships must be able to persist throughout necessary, productive conflict, culminating in deeper levels of communication and appreciation.

Friendship does not necessitate conflict, as long as friends find some ways to express their differences. Interpersonal tensions need not surface antagonistically, nor need they be resolved in order for a friendship to persist. Accepting people for who they are is essential to friendship, but we only fully accept others after we accept ourselves. In order to be a friend and have friends, it is essential that we gain increased self-acceptance from knowing and developing an identity of our choice.

The termination of a friendship may be necessary when a friend does not allow interpersonal differences to be acknowledged. Incapacity to discuss changes in communications or negotiations impedes the growth of both friends. Only friendships that can be worked on are ultimately in women's real interests. Women cannot afford to stand still in their lives. Their ability to move forward means progressing into stronger identity and friendships rather than perpetuating passive adaptation. Friendship is not gained or sustained easily, but rather crafted with effort and courage. Friendship is richest when it is deep.

## NEUTRALIZING ISOLATION

Friendship allows women to break out of isolating family roles. Meaningful, continuing contact with women outside their families fosters increased objectivity about domestic responsibilities. We see ourselves more clearly when we know how outsiders see us, and are more astute about our own lives when comparing our behavior with that of other women in similar circumstances.

Very close relationships may threaten us. We withdraw from emotional tightness and others' demands when we are in very intense, closed emotional systems. This withdrawal is an attempt to preserve self from the strong influence of those closest to us. The protective move further isolates us, however, and we cannot experience companionship. An irony is that being too close to family members prevents us from loving fully, spontaneously, or in ways that intellectually we would choose. Friendship builds bridges for women. Friendship allows women to be freer within traditional responsibilities and to move outside others' expectations. Friendship enables women to see a broader, more representative picture of the outside world. It is only when women get to know territory beyond family domains that they can cultivate meaningful autonomy for themselves. Women cannot select preferred options until they know that options exist.

Women who live and work in their own homes are more likely to be isolated than women who have contacts with a variety of people in different geographical or occupational locations. This segregation becomes less when women have meaningful friendships with each other. Women's attitudes towards themselves, community, and society are changed or even transformed through friendships.

Many of women's problems, such as lack of mobility and low self-esteem, arise from overcommitment to family responsibilities and overdependency on family members. Friendships show us a viable way out of this suffocation and inhibition of energies.

Identity increases our motivation to change all aspects of our lives. Identity necessitates seeing ourselves in connection with others rather than in isolation. Women become full participants in society and full participants in evolution by moving out of their domestic isolation. Exploration of values and alternative activities through the concern and attention of others is one of the most effective ways women have to break out of their isolation. Friendships promote enhanced personal awareness and women's social development. The reciprocal nurturing of women by women ultimately achieves broad social changes.

## CHOICES

Identity and behavior change according to the choices that women make. Women empower themselves through their decisions and active participation. Choices are possible only when options are discerned. Issues for consideration in decision-making about friendship are listed here.

1 Women must choose to extend themselves to others in order to break out of their isolation. Friendships are a significant and meaningful self-extension.

2 Family members have lifetime bonds with each other. By contrast, friends are transient, but they have the power to increase objectivity about self and family roles. Women need friendships that enable them to understand themselves.

3 Friends reflect our values or manifest values that we would like to have. Our choices of friends are crucial for clarifying our values.

4 We get to know who we want to be through our friendships. Our choices in friends increase our awareness of our possibilities.

5 As we clarify identity and modify major commitments, we tend to replace our friends. If we do not replace them, our friendships are eventually modified.

6 Social mobility includes making changes in our reference groups or in

our relationships with those who imbue our lives with special meaning. When we choose to raise our social status, we make new friends.

**7** When we choose to have friends we simultaneously choose to be friends. Ideally friendship is reciprocal. We must gain sustenance and inspiration from our friendships before we can give these to other women.

**8** We cherish our friendships most when we work on them by acknowledging and resolving personal differences. Choosing to ignore relationship issues means that a deterioration in the friendship will follow.

**9** Women's expertise in expressing nurturing values in family settings can be directed to friendships. We look after our best interests by cultivating nurturing friendships and nurturing self.

**10** Wherever we are we can choose to be friends with others. Friendships are both long-standing and transient, depending on our choices and needs. In all social contexts, we have much to gain from choosing to be a friend.

Chapter 12

# Community

Communities are complex systems of social exchanges or negotiations. Each member participates in communities at a level of integration of values and concerns that transcends individual interests. In return for subordinating singular to collective interests, communities provide their members with opportunities and goals for meaningful achievement.

We need communities in order to survive and we express ourselves most fully through our active participation in them. The quality of our involvement in our neighborhood and work communities sets the tone for other dimensions of our lives. When people are in harmony with their environment, they are more productive. The give and take of community living is more beneficial when we understand ourselves. Focusing on identity prompts us to develop our talents and to use them for the benefit of the collective.

Women need to participate actively in communities in order to establish more flexible relationships. Because it is more difficult for women to change their behavior solely within their own nuclear families, they can more readily neutralize the negative effects of traditional domestic roles within the context of community participation. These settings inspire increases in models and styles of identity. Political participation and professional activity redefine women's role options. Increasing numbers of women working outside the home now benefit from this directly, and community activity has diminished their isolation within domestic milieus. Through community participation women provide their children with socially oriented role models as an alternative to the endless generational repetitions of confined domestic roles.

New hope is born and nurtured within communities. However, women must begin with their own values and personal lives. Clinical data show that women's transitions to more conscious identity and more deliberate decisions potentially enhance the lives of all people. Value changes permit women to exercise more effective control of their own lives. By increasing their participation in the community women transform social structures into more open and equitable systems.

The quality of life cannot be legislated or mandated by societal leaders. Officials may remove obstacles, but in the long run individual responsibility and initiative are required to create, establish, and maintain a meaningful life. Clinical data show that fulfillment derives less from engagement at public and institutional levels, than from personal and community spheres.

While communities have traditionally been stratified to the advantage of men, widespread alienation has raised the challenge of building new communities with more equitable forms of power and influence. Family research suggests that increased equality among women and men engenders more flexible social control and more opportunities for participation. It appears that more enlightened planning can enhance life for all without restricting or impairing opportunities and activities.

Community is built on cooperation not competition and it encourages a large variety of member contributions. Though we cannot move readily from our current circumstances to an ideal community, we advance towards more satisfactory arrangements when we envisage the possibilities. Social inventions in human relations promise alternatives to those current structures that work only in the interests of a few. Letting go of the deeply ingrained, self-limiting conviction that women's subordination is inevitable is a prerequisite for new, more life-giving communities.


## PARTICIPATION

Though communities appear to have rigid hierarchies of power and material stratifications, they have an underlying dynamic of exchange and negotiation. Women's community participation patterns have generally been passive and veiled from public view. Equality with men requires changes in familial responsibilities to permit women's more active community involvement. As they increase their active community participation and equality, women achieve a more equitable partnership with men.

Cross-cultural research data show that although women have historically led busy and pressured lives, much of their activity has been channeled into traditional domestic roles rather than exploration, adventure, and risk-taking. It is only through awareness of identity and interests that women are able to direct their activities and community participation creatively and constructively.

Passive participation in communities predisposes women to be victims of circumstance. By being less than full participants in the community, women become less autonomous and less in charge of their own lives. Passivity is a retreat from life, and whether externally or internally imposed, leads to vulnerability and excessive attention to others' expectations and demands. There can be no fulfillment for women as silent partners to men's achievements. True liberation for women means freedom from social restrictions and freedom to engage fully in community activity.

Clinical data show that personal relationships and family bonds are enlivened and reinforced by women's increased community participation. Feminists believe that increased community activity by women does not necessarily diminish that of men, but instead generates a balance within community processes. When communities are burdened by imbalanced participation, their flexibility and life-enhancing qualities are reduced. Passivity generates conditions of alienation and extinction. Stagnant membership makes communities unable to adapt to broader social structures or to their own unfolding realities.

Through a lifetime of incremental choices women carve out their destinies. Independent women assume community and familial responsibilities, and their lives expand into the community through friendship networks. Such a broad arena for individual and social expression promotes individual and familial well-being, and ultimately transforms community structures.

Rapid social change has broken down and modified many of our established interrelational patterns, providing opportunities to build more equitable and fulfilling structures. Feminists believe that those communities are more viable which welcome equality of opportunity and equitable participation by all. Isolation in the family deprives women of opportunities for a richer life. Extension into the community ultimately connects women to the larger evolution and to a broader universe of meaning. More balanced community participation suggests many possibilities for change.

## FLEXIBILITY

Inflexibility is a serious malady in most extant social institutions. Ossification of social process stifles human creativity, and rigid gender roles promote sexism and dehumanization. Women are trapped in the static expectations of society's institutional core, and only more flexible roles and expectations can change women's personal and public lives.

Although significant changes in prevalent social institutions are so gradual as to seem impossible, community structures can be modified by shifts in participation patterns. Clinical data suggest that contemporary women are more motivated to change their behavior than are men. Thus, community transformations more frequently evolve from modifications in women's behavior. As women assume multiple roles outside the narrow range of domestic responsibilities, men also diversify their roles. Role diversification enhances options for both women and men.

More flexible role definitions and broader opportunities for community participation promote awareness of options, as women explore further afield in search of wholeness. Narrow role definitions stunt personal growth, while broader options urge women to experiment with identity empowerment. Historically women have been allowed very little mobility in community and family settings. Today, however, women are more aware of their options and thus more flexible in their responsiveness to both family and community needs.

Traditional roles persist in community structures and many women continue to choose them or follow them out of habit or custom. Flexibility suggests freer choices, not the elimination of particular roles or options. Although generational patterns are no longer repeated by all women, they may choose to uphold specific family traditions.

In modern societies women are not born into particular roles with the expectation that they will perform them throughout their lifetimes. Rather than accepting ascribed functions, they define and achieve roles. Through efforts to redefine and attain roles women modify traditional structures and in the process transform communities. The resultant flexibility in communities promotes qualitative changes in women's lives, including increased expansiveness in community living.

Women are moving from a caste to their own specific status. Flexibility in the community is achieved when women achieve status heterogeneity over inherited caste or functional class. Diversity, specialization, and the innate richness of human qualities create multiple and varied opportunities for accomplishment and self-expression in flexible communities. Until recently, women achieved status not in their own right but through their father's or husband's achievements. New options have generated sufficient structural change and flexibility in communities that women are recognized on their own merits. Women express themselves fully by contributing to community, and status is bestowed on them as social recognition for this contribution.

## RECIPROCITY

Community is a collective process characterized by reciprocal exchanges. It is the entity through which a wide range of values is expressed. When values are clearly defined and similar, there is less likelihood that conflict will occur. Though ambiguities or contradictions in values may lead to estrangement among community members, the vitality of the collective benefits from value heterogeneity.

Reciprocity characterizes successful relationships. It denotes return in kind for contributions made. An individual's action is valued, and thus prompts a similar response. Exchanges are not necessarily equal in this process, but it is believed that contributions made by each participant are of comparable worth. Interaction becomes a mutual negotiation wherein individuals seek maximum benefits without inordinate sacrifice. Before proffering specific services or goods, an individual assesses the others' willingness to negotiate. In the final analysis, we negotiate our most important values with each other.

Historically, women have tended to be locked into exploitative negotiations. Dependence and the need for acceptance by others stabilize patterns in exchanges whereby women give services, remain passive in decision-making, and are vulnerable to men. Both genders conceived of a reality where women's roles were quite narrowly defined. These patterns can be changed, however, when women are sufficiently motivated to reach out of their isolation and participate in community-level exchanges.

Reciprocity is not ours to choose. Our behavior is shaped by the mutual dependence of all, and without shared values we stand outside human discourse and civilization. Although value decisions are problematic and painful, shifts in traditional roles occur only when women reach out beyond their families and participate in their own right in the wider community.

Reciprocity creates predictable patterns or norms in social interaction. Changes in individual behavior have a direct impact on those around us, particularly within family milieus. In the early stages of women's empowerment, conflict and resistance are precipitated among those who stand to lose privileges by the advance of equality. Clinical data show an inverse relationship between dependence and conflict, that is, intense dependence precludes overt expressions of value dissension. Thus, increased interdependence brings a higher probability of conflict as women achieve the latitude to express their dissatisfaction with the status quo.

Liberation and empowerment mean increased autonomy for women in their relationships to men and other women, as well as in their choice of roles. Women have the responsibility to carve out their own destinies, a task qualitatively different from responding to traditional expectations and demands. Women gain control over their lives by deciding to act in their own interests. Empowerment means women's substitution of new definitions for their inherited and acquired patriarchal concepts of reality.

Mutual reciprocity reins in the individuating tendencies that have historically alienated women and diminished their collective strength. As women participate more fully in collective action, they acknowledge the strength of reciprocity in their lives. Collective action thus harmonizes women's individual interests.

Cross-cultural data show that women in industrialized countries are moving out of exchanges based on personal loyalty into broader patterns of reciprocity. This shift is manifested in society as transformed role definitions and mainstream values, and collective action opens the way for women to enjoy more expansive and effective lives. Community reciprocity facilitates the expression of women's individual and social protests about a status quo which restricts their life-chances.

## PRODUCTIVITY

Productivity is the extent to which we benefit one another in a community setting. Reciprocal exchanges and negotiations enhance and enrich our skills and enterprises, and we thrive individually and collectively by increasing our productivity.

Identity allows us to pursue our interests within reciprocal relationships and seek routes of even greater productivity. When we discover and assess our skills, our position is stronger than if we merely react to others' pressures and demands. We give most to others when we engage in activities which we enjoy.

As women clarify their identity and increase their community activity, they become more productive in both their private lives and the public sector. Enhanced community activity does not detract from full engagement in the domestic milieu. In fact, many women have found that the more valued their contribution to the community, the greater their willingness to give to family members. As increased productivity in the community enhances self-esteem, its impact is amplified in the other areas of our lives. Clinical data evidence that the broader our scope of participation, the more able and willing we are to give to those emotionally closest to us.

We are at our most productive when our relationships are balanced and harmonious. Peaceful environmental conditions increase the number and quality of our contributions. Patterns of dominance and submission are particularly deleterious to productivity, as they curtail freedom of expression and activity. Conflict, however, may be creative and conducive to a more profound and lasting harmony as it prompts social transformation. Because it so dramatically alters dependence patterns, conflict opens closed relationships and ultimately enhances interdependence.

Industrialization and modernization have led to increased pluralism and specialization. Communities are more diverse, as are their channels of productivity. As women move into roles outside their domestic milieus, overall productivity becomes even more diversified. Women's special kinds of productivity enrich community living. They have long dealt with various practical matters, such as child care and budgeting, and the transfer of these skills from the domestic milieu to occupational and professional roles is quite effective. As well as increasing abundance in productivity, women discover new and more practical ways of accomplishing tasks to meet individual and social needs. It can be surmised, then, that women's increased participation in the community will bring about increased production for all.

Women improve their occupational and professional skills by building working relationships with other women. Their productivity is increased and more fully appreciated through trading ideas and information with women who have similar interests. Networking nurtures self-confidence and mutual trust, as occupational exchanges move women beyond friendships into the larger world of business.

Women's productivity leads to economic independence and full partnership with men in domestic and social responsibilities. Their productivity also provides a model for children. Children see and learn that life has many purposes and directions, and that giving to others outside the family is important. Women's productivity changes their position in the community, consequently changing their families.

The results of women's talents and productivity speak for themselves. They bring recognition and rewards from the community. Women's genius in leadership and enterprise—for centuries hidden from public view—emerges and is expressed.

## COOPERATION

Women need other women in order to accomplish this transition from family to community. Interaction with friends and neighbors gives way to occupational networks and increased productivity. These patterns in women's relationships are characteristically cooperative. Women work together in order to free one another and to enrich each other's private and public lives.

Cooperative action is an expression of the nurturing values that most women have historically espoused as their own. Women's liberation articulates new and different values and recognizes selected traditional values as useful in expanding women's opportunities. Cooperation evolves from women's exchanges, founded on the necessity to support others' development of potential.

Traditionally, women have associated nurturing with dependent family members such as children and incapacitated older parents. Women have also nurtured their husbands, providing the background support necessary for men's occupational, geographical, and social mobility.

Whereas women have sustained cooperation to meet others' needs, men have been more preoccupied with competition. Competitive social processes and structure have evolved through men's dominance over women. Women's cooperative modes of relating to each other become more widespread as women participate more fully in community activity.

Women's full partnership with men balances cooperative and competitive modes in social relations. Such a balance is not merely life-enhancing but also life-saving. Imbalances and impasses have resulted from men's dominance and competitive styles of negotiations. By placing a stronger value on cooperation, we work more effectively as teams in our concerted efforts to reach collective goals. Competition denies the reality that we need each other.

Cooperation is the most effective behavioral expression of reciprocity. We express our innate interdependence when we work and live cooperatively with others. Rather than contending for the same material rewards and rivalry over limited resources so characteristic in competition, cooperation promotes greater respect for individual members' contributions to the whole.

Cooperation is a more rewarding negotiation; social relationships change when emphasis is given to joint efforts rather than competitive struggles. Friendship and occupational networks become viable bases or models for the development of qualitatively new kinds of cooperative communities.

Women's focus on identity prevents a loss of individual distinctiveness in cooperative effort. Identity ensures self-preservation in the face of others' needs. Further, identity harnesses and organizes energies directed to cooperative effort. Women need to define clearly their identity prior to transitions into communitywide cooperative enterprises.

Women are in the forefront of developing cooperation and of defining and refining identity. The awareness of innate equality that feminism has heightened needs to be cultivated and expressed in women's actions to make further advances. Men's awareness and behavior changes follow women's example. Unless there are marked shifts in women's activity at community levels, however, men will feel no need to change their competitive behavior.

## POSSIBILITIES

Women's progress in personal and public growth provides indicators of possibilities for society and civilization. Vision is necessary for women to translate ideals into action. Women's pioneering efforts serve not only their own interests, but men's as well. Though women may not be accepted by men as role models, their expansive values can inspire men's efforts to liberate themselves from various restrictions. Indeed, inspired by women, men may find the strength and motivation needed to discard confining roles and expectations.

Neither women nor men benefit from setting unattainable ideals. Women's individual and collective empowerment implies extending the realm of the possible rather than insisting upon the attainment of unrealistic goals. Women aim not for utopian perfection, but for broader more numerous opportunities for fulfillment. When women see one another taking charge of themselves and making substantial contributions to the community, their belief that they can successfully accomplish this is reconfirmed.

Within the context of community, many possibilities for women can be identified. Although women are not equally represented among world powers, they are attaining ever more significant societal positions. Grass-roots activities of women give momentum to increased opportunities for greater social advancement. Women's community activities are prototypes of possibilities for broader societal contributions.

Women's political activism in communities is easier to document than many other ways in which they work to change values and attitudes. Legislative processes have traditionally been dominated by men. It is difficult for women to enter political arenas and remain true to their own values and interests. Political activity exerts such a strong influence on women, however, that they are forced to internalize male values in order to survive the impact of political processes and to be heard by men in that context.

A review of their possibilities suggests that women transmit a variety of powerful influences rather than the narrow range of political power defined by men. Although women may not become official religious leaders, for example, they may actually be the spiritual leaders of particular religious groups. The kinds of power women provide become increasingly evident as they participate in community and societal change.

One of the central issues in women's growth, development, and liberation is their assumption of personal and public power. By assuming more varied responsibilities and wielding their more cooperative values, women move out of powerlessness. Identity is a means of becoming more powerful as it releases women from the entrapments of passivity and apathy. By breaking out of socially imposed isolation, women find each other, and through that contact empower themselves. Demonstrations of the power of collective action and identity empowerment increase women's motivation to make further changes on behalf of those who still live as victims at the brink of despair.

Possibilities for women flow from their power. While others may not recognize women as having power in their own right, women's advancement enables them to escape social paralysis and make effective social changes. Nurturing values express women's power, and society is regenerated through their application. Tolerance and respect are increased through women's power. Women's values are inclusive and more towards harmony, not towards competition and divisiveness. To the extent that women achieve full partnership with men through community action, society generates new creative synthesis and balance.

## GENERALIZATIONS AND PROPOSITIONS

Women's search for identity and their expression of identity through community actions suggest a number of generalizations. Identity is both personal and social; self-discovery comes from knowing our individual preferences and aligning ourselves with the particular community values and social causes most likely to bring their realization.

Communities provide a middle-range perspective through which people can better understand themselves and society. Women's efforts to move into broader social arenas are described here.

1   Women's friendships are an empowering medium through which they move towards occupational networks and communities.

2   Women participate in community processes by deciding to be active and by refusing to perpetuate passive roles.

3   Through their efforts to interact as equals, women establish full partnership with men in communities.

4   Flexibility in roles allows women to change their community participation patterns. Survival requires significant modifications of rigid social institutions.

5   Reciprocity can be shifted into productive relations based on cooperative not competitive community exchanges. Women's experience is particularly conducive to promoting meaningful reciprocity and cooperation.

6   Women's community activities create new syntheses in broader social change.

7   Women's pioneering efforts in community participation serve as models for the future. Men and children learn from the expression of women's values in action.

Propositions specify particular relationships among these generalizations and trends. Although clinical and life-history data about women's changes are sparse, some pertinent questions and issues can be outlined.

1   The grass-roots empowerment of women eventually brings about community change. Women increase their possibilities and probabilities for social effectiveness to the extent that they identify themselves with power.

2   Women's nurturing values promote cooperation, increased role flexibility, and more supportive reciprocity.

3   Cooperative efforts promote long-run productivity and increasingly diverse community output.

4   Identity gives women a foundation for their own uniqueness with respect to collective action. Identity prevents the merging of self into reciprocal and cooperative engagements.

5   Community is a meaningful and effective arena for the expression of

identity and cooperation. Whatever their personal or professional accomplishments, all women are needed in grass-roots efforts to open new frontiers.

**6** The need for more equal relations between women and men motivates women to exercise different types of power. To the extent that women believe that they have power, and find areas in which to exercise it, they are better able to abandon restrictive roles.

**7** Community interaction illustrates the process through which women transfer their energies, skills and experiences from the domestic milieu to broader spheres. By identifying with particular values, women are motivated to expand their roles and activities.

# Chapter 13

# Transcendence

Transcendence is an affirmation of our ideals and values. The ability to see beyond difficult living conditions or harsh circumstances is not restricted to a spiritually endowed elite. Transcendence is contemplation and reflection that enable us to see beyond immediate appearances.

Transcendence is consciousness that results from attention to meaningful values or ideals. Investment in values of long-term significance gives direction to decisions and order to priorities. Transcendence is sustained more easily when values are fairly consistent and stable, as such coherence is essential for endurance. Our activities must be coordinated if they are to be effective and have an impact on others.

Transcendence is a means for women to focus on their possibilities and long-range goals rather than on restricted circumstances and existing hardships. Women transcend their limited self-concepts when they express their real interests.

Transcendence harnesses energies. Women must step back from difficult or complex conditions in order to understand and reflect upon the significance of their choices in those circumstances. This is purposeful retreat, and a new view of one's life and sense of identity is created through transcendence.

Women cultivate habits of transcending everyday routine to get more in control of their lives, and to be better able to see their available choices. Transcendence is a way to put oneself in the universe, to see purpose in one's life in light of the broadest and deepest concerns. Women are able to define themselves more powerfully when they turn to values which go beyond themselves.

Transcendence enhances personal relationships and capacities to cope with general living conditions. This process or state of being diminishes our dependence on intimates, and thus puts breathing space into our personal relationships. Exchanges between two people are more harmonious when each individual is emotionally invested in transcendent values. When attention is given to one's own ideals, thoughts, and feelings, others are not perceived as threats or competitors.

Personal or social crises are opportunities to increase our capacities to transcend our reactivity and limited self-concepts. At these times our deepest, most cherished values are shaken, and we make sense of our lives only by seeing ourselves differently. When we have a deeper understanding of who we are, we develop spiritual faculties as guides in our decision-making and selection of new goals.

Transcendence is a kind of prayer and meditation. By turning our attention to ideals of love, trust, harmony, or peace, we detach ourselves from the immediate demands of others. This transcendence is not withdrawal since ideals frequently include participation and action.

Transcendence allows us to be honest with ourselves. We understand what we are doing with our lives only when we detach from our emotional involvement with others. We love more fully when we loosen our possessiveness. We are less enslaved by others when we transcend annoying or petty conditions in our personal relationships.

Transcendence does not necessitate ignoring others' definitions of reality. We need to stay in touch with shared perceptions, but this should be contact, not conformity. We cannot live exclusively in our own worlds, and we must acknowledge conventional meanings.

We transcend limitations in our lives and others' demands by selecting values meaningful to us. Objectivity comes from strengthening our capacity to transcend our existing situations. We come into our own only by becoming more objective about life.

## IDENTITY

Identity is a mechanism through which we link physical, emotional, mental, and transcendental levels of self. Transcendental self generates motivation to attain these ideals. Transcendence is a level of experience which enables us to consolidate and integrate identity.

Life is transformed when transcendent values, such as trust and knowledge, become more important than pleasing others through traditional role-playing. Individuality is expressed more freely through our deliberate choices of ideals and values than in role behavior. Identity integrates physical, mental, and emotional realities with spiritual possibilities, and transcendent values become a dominant influence on action and commitments.

Identity anchors us in social institutions through our choice of durable values. Institutional values transcend idiosyncrasy. All human beings are traditional to the extent that they internalize established values in order to be functioning members of society. Identity calls imagination into play—we are what others perceive us to be, and also what we perceive ourselves to be. When we strengthen the idealistic component of identity, we transcend others' perceptions and seize our own destinies. We become more than what others see us to be by articulating our ideals in identity. Ideals are key means of transcending our restricted roles and limited goals.

Self is expressed more clearly and more decisively through identification with powers such as justice, truth, or nature. Women become more motivated to work their way through many of the inhibiting complexities of their lives when they identify with some power beyond themselves. Self-alignment with power through identity animates spirit and energy and enables women to break through passivity to activity. When they do not idealize a form of power, women remain programmed to lead more withdrawn, invisibly active lives of nurturing and supporting others.

Identity allows us to transcend everyday realities, however harsh those realities may be. Identity oriented towards our strongest ideals and values focuses our attention on possibilities rather than on problems. This is not a false hope; recognize, however, that ideals do not deny harmful conditions in our lives. Ideals allow us to direct our energies into more constructive, creative channels. It is more soothing and fulfilling to see what we can do with our lives than to emphasize binding restrictions.

Identity becomes balanced through the integration of the facts of our lives and ideals. Until recently women valued traditional roles that met others' expectations rather than formulating and achieving their own ideals. Responsibility includes discerning higher purposes in life as well as meeting practical needs for survival. Women involved in this revolution are daring to select goals of their own and work towards them. This effort is transcendence, linking identity to past, present, and future ideals and values.

## IDEALS AND COMMITMENT

Ideals are the essence of identity and the substance of our values. Historically, women harbored very few ideals of their own. Socially endorsed ideals for women are only aspects of their central obligation to care for others and disregard self. Education opens the world of women, however, enabling them to entertain a variety of ideals transcending traditional roles.

Ideals go beyond present empirical realities, establishing links with the past and future. They allow women to imagine a heaven on earth, and gives them a vision on which to build their own utopia. Ideals and commitments are a motivating force in women's lives, but only after they select ideals can they make meaningful, lasting commitments. Progressive changes occur when women incorporate their chosen ideals in daily activity.

Transcendence through ideals and commitments empowers women to deal with current problems, issues, and goals. Having ideals and commitments makes them less reactive to others' demands, and at the same time better able to respond to their real needs. Reactivity ultimately blocks communication with others, and inhibits the ability to give. When women invest attention and energy in ideals which transcend current settings, they are more fulfilled and find meaning in meeting requests. In this way we are all civilized through ideals and commitments that elevate us beyond irritations and aggravations in daily interaction.

Women see a larger world through empowering identity. They establish contact with a broader range of ideals than restrictive domestic milieus allow. By selecting specific ideals as their own, and through making commitments to put these into action, women transcend some of the boundaries of their lives, such as their own and others' expectations. Transcendence puts individuals and groups in contact with a moral power that has the potential to overturn political power.

By embracing equality as an ideal, women make more effective commitments to bring equality to all aspects of their personal and public lives. Their vision of equality, and use of equality as a source of inspiration and action, increases the moral power of equality in society. Moral power is the substance of values and attitudes which support or destroy the exercise of political power. Moral power neutralizes the effects of political power because political power cannot indefinitely overturn moral power. Clinical data show that when women's values and actions are aligned with universal truths, their moral force is indomitable.

Women's fulfillment is achieved only through incorporating more expansive ideals into their lives. Unless women select broad values characteristic of many kinds of people, their existence will be ghettolike, segregated, and confined to a low caste position. Evolution and life broaden rather than restrict experience, and ideals that converge on fulfillment develop the potential of women more than ideals which center on survival. Fulfillment transcends repetitions and drabness in our lives, moving us beyond the present to a more livable future. Growth and development through identity empowerment are spurred by transcendence, ultimately becoming metamorphosis.

## EMPOWERMENT

Empowerment results from aligning ourselves with forces beyond ourselves. We empower self by networking with others and by espousing values which transcend our limitations. Thus, we are empowered to the extent that we reach out effectively to other people and sources of strength.

Detaching from others allows us to be more autonomous and empowered. When we make our own decisions, we free ourselves from others' possessiveness and are able to give fully. The greater our empowerment, the greater the contribution we make.

The issue of power is central to women's equality. Historically, women's lives have been remote from the social sources of power. Powerlessness strongly influences women's definitions of reality—men have wielded power and women have experienced powerlessness. Women must cultivate a sense of power to break out of isolation and subordination.

Self-awareness and awareness that one is separate from those who are emotionally closest are the initial stages of women's empowerment. Self-awareness is a foundation of women's freedom, and may become a foundation for peace when sufficient numbers of women are empowered. Women's valuing their equality is essential to the ability to transcend injustices and inequality. At the same time this enables women to achieve equality in all social relations. Only when women deliberately empower themselves through transcendence can they achieve equality.

Transcendence is a stronger influence on behavior than the human will. Honoring values and striving towards selected ideals carries us beyond realms of rational calculation, even when initial choices of values and ideals are reasoned. Transcendence empowers us to see and act for the collective welfare. Women come to understand that their personal troubles are social issues which require dedicated commitment for resolution.

We can consciously cultivate mental, emotional, and spiritual states of transcendence. As our ability to do this is increased through practice, transcendence may be thought of as a skill. The cultivation of transcendence can be an end in itself, particularly to meet spiritual needs. Transcendence may also be a tool to empower individuals and groups, and a means to promote broad social change. Transcendence is an agent of empowerment; it puts us in touch with vital inner resources and life itself.

Consolidation or integration of self through identity allows us to delineate clearer senses of direction and purpose. We empower self when we transcend limitations in our present situations and move in a direction with purpose. Through transcendence we actualize our potential.

Empowerment and transcendence are processes. We grow in moral stature through our deliberate cultivation and encouragement of these processes in our lives. When we make empowerment central to us, we are empowered and work more effectively both alone and with others. In order to sustain our power, we must participate in the empowerment of others. Empowerment is not an achievement devoid of responsibilities. We only enhance our lives through empowerment when we have the interests of all at heart. If we abuse our privilege of power, we create new imbalances in social relations, destroying our ideal of equality as well as ourselves.

## CAUSE

A cause is a socially defined issue supported by people who press for changes in a specified direction. Women become militant or reformist through acting collectively to achieve equal rights in the whole population. Feminist causes are international in scope, as the plight of the majority of women in the world results from similar social conditions and attitudes.

The cause for equal rights allows women to transcend self and direct their energies toward broad goals of change. Women transcend personal needs and participate in community action. Alignment with feminism adds purpose and direction to the lives of individual women. It allows them to express their anger about their own and others' unjust suffering and despair in socially recognized ways.

However, transcendence through commitment to the cause of equal rights must be balanced by some focus on personal values and needs. Women cannot afford to move out of their subordination to men only to advance into new kinds of subordination to women who do not let them be themselves. Transcendence must be chosen rather than imposed or coerced, and tempered somewhat by the actualities and demands of living.

A cause requires many different kinds and levels of participation and accomplishment. Essential grass roots activity in a cause or social movement results from the hierarchies of values that individuals hold dear. Causes have their own priorities. The recognition, by participants, of varied value emphases within a particular cause may change the tenacity with which a person adheres to their own values. Women have begun to value power and its broad range of diverse manifestations through their participation in the cause for equal rights.

A cause is a current of history, a surge of revolutionary and evolutionary tides. The feminist movement shifts through time and sweeps women along in its cause for equal rights. The cause transforms private lives into social concerns in public arenas.

Women go beyond themselves in a cause—beyond their own life spans, and beyond their self-concepts and world views. Individual and social transcendence elevate aspirations and morale, and women are able to achieve more as a group than they could alone. Participation in a cause boosts individuals and may uplift society.

A cause moves in a specific direction and may have only one primary goal. A single legislative change, like the Equal Rights Amendment, has the power to galvanize an entire social movement. In reality, however, even single-goal causes carry with them multiple related issues. Causes promote change. Once the primary goal is accomplished, further changes occur in its wake.

A cause requires commitment and deliberate support from followers. Participation in a cause is reduced to conformity when the cause becomes an established social movement or an institutionalized change. The cause loses its militant appeal at this stage of widespread acceptance, as well as most of its power to transcend individual and group goals. The cause cannot be a means of transcendence when it is taken for granted. New causes emerge and gain power to transcend empirical realities. They elevate participants through transcendence and give them a sense of participating in eternal life.

## UNITY

Transcendence and participation in a cause heighten our unity with others. Actions within the women's cause help them to know that they are not only an integral part of the women's movement, but also part of the human race. By recognizing their own real interests women transcend their personal self, unite with other women, and unite with society as a whole. A paradox is that women experience their uniqueness more fully through identifying with life—with the whole of society, with history or with evolution—than they do by living in their roles.

Uniting with people who have the same or similar interests gives women increased strength to combat existing conditions. Women transcend their idiosyncratic selves through unity, and discover concerns that apply to all. Women's unity is a symbol of transcendence.

Unity of purpose creates group identity. By establishing collective goals for action, women's concerted efforts take on specific characteristics. Group values closely resemble individual participants' values, but in some cases group unity is achieved in spite of major individual differences.

The women's movement cannot realistically aspire to unite all women through the same priorities. The unity of women must necessarily be heterogeneous because pluralism is an integral part of modern industrial society. Women transcend self by uniting with other women to accomplish a specific cause. However, women also need to remain true to their own perceptions of reality and to their own values. Although unity among women is a precondition for effective collective action, it cannot be allowed to suffocate individual differences. The women's movement is a vital force for constructive change through pluralistic unity. Women need to both transcend and consolidate self. Identity allows them to do this by embracing individual differences and sharing social values and concerns.

Women unite with each other through their real interests. Women also unite with men through their shared claims to the good life. All people unite with life in the universe through the conditions of their existence. Our right to live fully on life's terms preserves and develops our lives.

Our innate affinity with these broadest concerns puts us more fully in touch with life and at the same time empowers us. When we realize that our spirits are part of an eternal Life Force, we are empowered. We become inspired through our unity with life, love, good, or truth, and as a consequence are able to transcend blocks in our personal lives.

Our identification with other women liberates women's spirit. We may choose to participate in a universal religion, such as Judaism or Christianity, but we may find that some religious beliefs inhibit rather than promote transcendence. This is especially apparent for women. We need to acquire energy and resources through unity with others, and not join in rigid rituals or traditional observances. To the extent that Judaism or Christianity are both unifying and liberating influences, they express both women's individual and collective interests.

The quality of unity within the women's movement influences the effectiveness of collective action and the number of opportunities for individual women. Human beings are dependent on society for their survival, and individual women's choices are dependent on the options available to women as a whole. Individual women may transcend limitations imposed on all women, but individual women are not able to change the lot of all women. Unity is a prerequisite for enhancing women's identity, commitments, and empowerment.

## CHOICES AND CHANGE

Individuals cannot escape their destiny as historical actors. Whether women choose to be active or passive, they are agents of change. Even if women are physically imprisoned or physically coerced, they have options and cannot escape the burden or opportunity of choice. We express ourselves through our choices, and we have a direct impact on change through our choices.

Our ability to transcend empirical realities exerts a powerful influence on our decision-making. If we see beyond the present with an awareness and understanding of the past, we can direct our activity towards a more productive, more fulfilling future. If we remain rooted in current circumstances without any substantial degree of transcendence, we make only short-run, unenlightened decisions.

Each choice expresses values we hold. We cannot escape value judgments in decision-making, nor can we avoid making choices. To the extent that we transcend the here and now of our lives and see the broader picture of life, we are free of social conditioning and restrictive roles.

One of women's significant choices is whether to move in the direction of survival or fulfillment. Either we decide to perpetuate the status quo by repeating past behavior or we enhance our lives by pioneering in the development of our potential. To the extent that we contribute directly to society as a whole, we achieve increased recognition and fulfillment.

Women's decision to perpetuate the status quo generally leads towards their further impairment. When change promotes growth and empowers women, it leads towards life rather than death. Ultimately, our choices settle around the fundamental issue of whether we want to live or die.

Our choices must be inclusive if we are to improve the quality of life for all. Women cannot exploit men in their progress towards equal rights. They must organize around the goal of full partnership with men in the creation, productivity, and governance of society. One of the most significant social transformations intended through the women's movement is to create conditions in which all live fully and celebrate life.

Issues of change revolve around our ideals, our visions of society and human nature, and our perceptions of life and the universe. Definitions of self and reality are permeated by and constructed from values. We are not victims of our values, however. We are free to select which values to emphasize in identity and commitments.

Transcendence is an important consideration in making value choices, and certain values help us to transcend difficult life situations more easily and effectively than others. Transcendent values such as justice promote the most dramatic changes of the status quo. Limited values, such as traditional definitions of femininity, inhibit change and impede the clarity and empowerment of identity.

## GENERALIZATIONS AND PROPOSITIONS

Transcendence is difficult to define and even more difficult to measure. Basic characteristics of transcendence highlight the nature of this process and its consequences for women as it is expressed in daily activity. The following selected generalizations relate particularly to women's experience.

1  Transcendence elevates women's point of view so they see the whole picture rather than the minutiae of interpersonal exchanges.

2  Transcendence increases women's objectivity, enabling them to detach from the possessive demands and expectations of those emotionally closest to them.

3  Transcendence is a useful skill for women to cultivate. An effective method to practice transcendence is to identify with ideals that reflect autonomy, integrity, and real interests, and not tradition or precedent.

**4** Transcendence links past, present, and future in meaningful ways, precipitating action to integrate these different time dimensions.

**5** Transcendence empowers women, especially those who participate in a social movement like feminism. Submerging personal values in goal-oriented ideals, such as equal rights for women, increases motivation to transcend existing boundaries in one's life and promotes the advancement of these ideals.

**6** Transcendence is a component of identity which consolidates values through the articulation of ideals.

**7** Transcendence develops through uniting with those who have similar interests. Transcendence inspires each person to go beyond limited personal interests.

Propositions link the properties of transcendence to the particular case of women and women's liberation. Transcendence is a dynamic of change, and influences the kind of change that occurs in women's lives. These propositions follow.

**1** To the extent that individual women transcend difficulties inherent in their life situations, they are able to increase their autonomy and improve the living conditions of other women.

**2** To the extent that groups of women transcend traditional expectations and role demands, they are able to promote substantive social change for equality and an overall enhancement of women's lives in society.

**3** Transcendence crystallizes empowerment efforts and promotes unity among women and between women and men.

**4** Ultimately women choose either to transcend self and embrace life, or to accept empirical realities and perpetuate patterns of conformity.

**5** Women transcend self by seeing their lives in the context of society and evolution, and by deciding to be historical actors.

**6** Values in women's identity are refocused by transcendental ideals. To the extent that women give their attention to ideals such as equality, their new perceptions and behavior transform their lives and promote marked social changes.

**7** The essence of women's grass-roots activism is the deliberate cultivation of transcendent ideals. Women are more energized for social and political activity towards equal rights if they focus their attention on transcendent ideals, such as freedom and justice, than if they give their attention to limitations and inequalities.

# Chapter 14

# Going Home

Home symbolizes domesticity, family roles, and female responsibilities. Women's roles in the home are historically circumscribed daily activities and life-course decisions. Indeed, the home has long been the primary site of oppression for women.

Women do not need to become dominant in domestic decision-making, but rather to participate equally in this process. They need to live comfortably and effectively in their homes, without being trapped in limiting roles. Women become victims of circumstance by accepting subordination as unavoidable. However, through identity empowerment they free themselves from burdensome, sometimes crippling demands related to family living. In these circumstances home is transformed from site of oppression to source of strength.

Women go home to retreat from the world and escape the stresses of broader challenges. When they repeat the domestic behavior patterns of past generations of women, however, they maintain the status quo. Ideally, women should go home to find themselves, replenish their energies, and size up opportunities and choices in their lives. Rather than going home and submitting to others' needs and demands, they can go home to plan action in the outside world.

Home is considered to be the foundation of our lives. Going home can be a means to make progress. When women go home to examine the source of their being, they reemerge with increased strength and enthusiasm for full living. They go home in order to advance.

Going home increases women's interest and ability to understand their roots. They know themselves more fully by looking at the different roles they perform in their families. By examining ways in which families interact, women become less likely to repeat patterns of subordination transmitted through generations.

Although going home means different things to various people depending on the degree of their awareness, this activity is universal. Both women and men gain much from a willingness to scrutinize their private lives and characteristic approaches to interaction. In times of rapid social change, members of the professional middle classes emphasize their public rather than private lives. However, in order to traverse the ambiguities of change, we must focus on the shared human condition when we go home to distance ourselves from the hurly-burly of everyday life.

Going home may be compared with observing a sabbath. We get a clearer sense of ultimate concerns in our lives when we retreat regularly and temporarily to our home bases. Going home may also be associated with reflection about the end of our lives. We try to achieve certain goals in our lifetime in order to have peace of mind. We set ourselves tasks to accomplish and go home when these are accomplished.

Going home is a way to contact sources of our own power and potential. Unless we retreat from mundane pursuits on a regular basis, we become wanderers. We need to know what our territory is in order to advance and enjoy full and effective lives.

We live in a fragmented world which depletes our energy. In spiritual terms, going home can be communing with nature, as we go home to connect ourselves with the greater powers of the universe. Through this kind of wholeness and oneness with others and the universe women and men are at home and themselves.


## SOURCE OF WELL–BEING

Ideally the home is a private sanctuary, a source of relaxation and well-being. All too often, however, domestic relations are combative. The home becomes an arena for dispute where energies are dissipated and sometimes destructive.

We create homes that directly reflect our deepest values and yearnings. The word *home* abounds with symbolic meaning. Although we may not be able to beautify our surroundings, home is a familiar place where we choose to be.

Traditionally, most of women's work has been performed at, or close to, home. As women's work options increase, they move away from their homes to exercise their skills and competence. Still, women's work generally encompasses responsibilities both inside and outside the home. This characteristic distinguishes women's work from men's work, which continues to be viewed as primarily outside the home.

Thus, women's rebellion and revolution lie in their refusal to dissipate their energies at home. Women need a refuge from their new community demands. The home must promote women's well-being, not place inordinate demands and stress on them. It is essential and necessary, not a luxury, for women to replenish their energies at home.

Women's redefinition of home as source of well-being is not easily accomplished. Others' expectations are neutralized only by women's concentrated efforts to give priority to their need for temporary withdrawal from society and time to reflect. Women must make time for themselves in order to survive and be fulfilled. When they value being home for the purposes of nurturing themselves, home is a haven for women's regeneration of strength.

Women's traditional roles dictate that at home they are available to serve others. Historically women have dedicated their lives to their families, while other family members come and go. As women leave home more frequently and regularly, deeply entrenched patterns of behavior change. At the same time, however, many traditional expectations remain. Increases in women's work in the outside world have not replaced expectations that they should be available to serve family members' needs as before. Only women's resistance to others' refusals to accept their autonomy creates conditions where women experience home as source of well-being.

Home symbolizes a return to roots, foundation, and emotional reserves. Women's experience of being trapped in domestic roles makes it difficult for them to be at home in relaxed ways. The demands women associate with home neutralize many restful aspects of home. Negative associations can be broken only by women's continuous attempts to perceive differently the value of their having their own territory in the world.

Women's comfort in their own homes results from their coming full circle in the development of self. When women choose to be at home for their own purposes, they claim freedom within and from traditional roles and responsibilities. Women go home not only to retreat, but also to formulate strategies for more effective participation in the world. If women are effectively empowered when they are home, homes are entered as fully as they are left and left as fully as they are entered. In and of themselves, domestic milieus no longer define women's possibilities.

## SALVATION NOT OPPRESSION

Salvation comes with women's redefinition of their home territories and personal and family relationships. Women live in harmony with their souls when they center their lives more fully on their own interests. If women's actions are only reactions to the push and pull of others' demands, their lives cannot be meaningful or satisfying. Hope lies in knowing that women can transform their domestic oppression. The means of their entrapment become means of their salvation. Women clarify their identity and commitments by redefining their roles as woman, wife, and mother.

In order to empower their status at home, women must have some awareness of possibilities for freedom. Women can neutralize oppression only after they confront the conditions of their subordination. They move towards liberation and salvation when they recognize and deal with restrictions in their present situations.

There are many nuances and subtleties in the complex variety of means of oppression, and it is not easy for women to delineate all of the ways in which they are oppressed. Generally speaking, it is only when women experience their oppression as pain or personal troubles that they are sufficiently motivated to make changes that lead them towards fuller living or salvation.

Women's personal lives are political. Power plays between women and men arise in the guise of issues in daily routines. Territorial rights are viewed as sacred and daily stresses revolve around scarce resources such as economic assets, time, and energy. Particularly in two-career households, women and men vie for who will or, more in fact, who will not perform particular chores. Disputes over the division of labor may supplant concerns about finances. When two incomes relieve economic needs, couples dispute other shared responsibilities.

Women must carve out their rights and responsibilities in domestic matters to be autonomous. They cannot afford to accept traditional feminine roles unquestioningly if these are not rewarding in the long run. Many women and men choose to have families to meet their needs for intimacy and companionship. However, unless women are alert to the influence of the wide range of oppressive forces that flow from this decision, they are trapped and unable to live their own lives.

Thus, the home may be thought of as a laboratory for self-strengthening. Women must negate, or at least neutralize, all the patterns that have produced oppression. Achieving this goal in domestic milieus is a crucial step, but do not underestimate the task—women's salvation is not won easily.

## CONSOLIDATING ENERGIES

Fragmentation is a disastrous consequence of the stresses in women's lives. Contributions to the community require integrated efforts and purposeful direction. Going home allows women to gather their strength for action. Once women's distractions are put aside, the home becomes a haven for cultivating a closer relationship with the self.

Women are conditioned to organize their lives around family needs. While they are not in the habit of using their home as a place in which to relax and rest, taking time for themselves in familiar surroundings is a constructive way for women to consolidate their energies. Recuperation is necessary to clarify identity and formulate plans.

Women's subordination and alienation have severed their contacts with power. In general, women have been excluded from opportunities to pursue and wield political and economic power. What political and economic privileges women have enjoyed have generally been those acquired from fathers and husbands.

Modern society allows a small percentage of women to have some political and economic power, usually at local levels. By consolidating their energies, women increase their access to diverse forms of power. Women can also capitalize on the skills they acquire through participating in family, religion, and education. Going home becomes a deliberate act to facilitate their recuperation of energy for developing strategies to contribute to society. Broader social participation minimizes women's powerlessness and maximizes their power.

Another aspect of consolidating energies in the home milieu is the practice of changing the patterns in which women relate to others. They can continue to respond to relatives' needs through activities that are less enervating than traditional nurturing functions. Others' demands are viewed from a new perspective when consolidating energy becomes a high priority for women. By attending to their own needs as the basis of their productive living, women give in more selective and more meaningful ways. Saying no to certain requests is justified and more appropriate than sacrificing the self for any request. Energy is consolidated more effectively when actions are weighed and measured in light of their possibilities for long-term constructive contributions. Giving should enhance not deplete oneself.

## REFLECTION

Reflection plays a crucial role throughout different kinds of identity shifts. In our personal lives and in society, inner transformation precedes significant external changes. Identity formulation directs and accomplishes change in attitudes towards oneself and others.

Reflection is at the heart of identity awareness and grass-roots activism. Enlightened action flows from the ability to consider alternatives. Inspired contributions and deeper levels of understanding result from creative reflection. Women become more objective about their skills and opportunities through reflection.

Contemplation in home surroundings promotes a relaxed attitude, which is conducive to understanding power. It increases our potential to see the broader picture of our lives. Although it may be difficult for many women to find peace and quiet in their homes, it is worth the effort to create an atmosphere for reflection.

Self-knowledge, planning, and goals evolve from reflection. Women break through fragmentation and compartmentalization in their lives by striving for wholeness in their daily activities. Regular reflection brings women into contact with the deepest parts of themselves and enables them to sustain a broader perspective on their lives.

Reflection may be both directed and undirected. In receptive reflection we contemplate selected ideas. Observing our thoughts and feelings makes our action more deliberate. Claiming enough time and privacy for reflection helps to overcome passivity.

Reflection must become a habit if women are to empower themselves. Clinical data confirm that it is easy for people—especially women—to let a decade go by without any consistent evaluation of responsibilities, contributions, and possibilities. Reflection ensures that our lives remain in a direction chosen by us, not set by others.

Going home to reflect imbues women's traditional domestic lives with new dimensions of meaning. Rather than home being the primary site of oppression, it becomes an incubator for women's freedom. When women go home to their parents, perhaps even to the home where they were raised, they are reconnected with their deepest roots. This experience deepens reflection, adding valuable time frames and depth of vision which cannot be part of their more routine reflections in their own homes.

Sometimes our greatest insights dawn while we are in the midst of simple activities. Inner reviews of action during the day transform women's activities, and dropping off to sleep is a productive period for syntheses. Women's goal is to apply their own standards to a thorough examination of their lives.

## PEACE

Peace of mind may be the ultimate objective of expressing identity in women's private and public lives. Peace of mind comes from knowing that one's actions are constructive activity.

Peace of mind can be worked on and peace in the world visualized in a home environment. Withdrawal from social roles may be women's only opportunity to see how things could be. Women may make substantial contributions to world peace. Clinical data show that they add nurturing values to perceptions and definitions of current situations, and to ways in which conflict is resolved or regulated.

Equality is an essential precondition but not the sole reason for the inclusion of women at all levels of decision-making. Equality sets the stage for full partnership between women and men in diverse tasks. Equality facilitates enlightened action and is not a complete activity in its own right. A major benefit of women's equal participation could be to bring new values to bear on our quest for world peace. Feminists speculate that world peace is more likely to occur when equality of opportunity and cooperation are institutionalized in mainstream society. Peace is precluded by the systematic discrimination and coercive subordination of certain segments of society. We need breakthroughs in our perceptions and thinking about survival in today's world.

Traditional roles have programmed women to be family peacemakers, and women's adeptness in mediation and arbitration is much needed. As women learn more about themselves, accepting and using their talents to a greater extent, they apply their negotiating skills in an increasingly wider range of social settings.

Women have peace of mind only when they give directly to the world at large. The freshness of women's vision enlivens peace efforts, and may ultimately lead to global survival. Women have been trained to be loving and caring, and this skill bolsters cooperative efforts for world peace.

Women's inner peace from fulfillment increases the possibility of external peace in society. Women may have to enter into conflict with others, however, before they can reach deep peace within themselves, their community, and society.

Thus, going home sets the stage for world peace movements within ourselves and in society. Male culture has not produced world peace. Patriarchies have led to a large number of social contradictions and imbalances, such as the hoarding of weapons for defense purposes. Female values—equality, cooperation, loving support, and caring for others—have a greater potential for restoring social balance, giving drive and direction to both internal and external peace efforts.

## RETREAT

Women retreat in order to prepare for constructive action. They purposefully retreat from the world but not from themselves or from their social responsibilities. Women go home so they can spring back into social life more effectively.

Regularly retreating from their involvement with others allows women to enter deliberately into a pendulum rhythm of invisible and visible activity. Women retreat in order to advance, and they advance more effectively as a result of that retreat. Retreat is necessary for women's survival and fulfillment, as it increases their participation in community and society. Even though retreat may be infrequent, like the observation of a weekly sabbath, regular retreat cannot be omitted without setting destructive consequences in motion. Retreat is not a stage in women's lives, but a regular observance that increases effectiveness in accomplishing their goals.

Women's retreat creates a new world. Whether active or passive, retreat pulls women out of the mainstream of public activity for a limited time. When retreat is chosen rather than imposed, women's home life is animated and transformed by their experience in the outside world.

Retreat balances public and private aspects of women's lives. It facilitates identity formulation, making commitments, and the consolidation of energies. Retreat promotes social action, increasing enthusiasm and interest in daily activity. Our speeds and emotional intensity must be deliberately paced if we are to accomplish our goals.

Retreat moves us back into our own resources and home becomes a haven from the world. It legitimizes detachment from others and from our work in the community. By making a deliberate effort not to do things, we stand still and let action happen through and beyond us.

Retreat allows women to see themselves for who they are. They can be honest about their own thoughts and feelings when they take them seriously and make an effort to know and understand them. They are not able to come to grips with who they are if they allow themselves to be continually submerged in activity.

Retreat enables women to examine their lives. They will not be able to live at fulfillment levels unless they formulate imaginative solutions to perplexing situations. Home becomes the retreat that allows them to value their direct contributions to society and their own lives. Women cannot live productively or think creatively when they are overburdened.

Retreat further enables women to participate more fully in history as they are in charge of the momentum of their lives. By withdrawing from activity, they become better able to move themselves forward through fuller self-expression. Going home begins and ends in action.

## CHOICES

Several strategies can change women's perceptions of the home from its traditional image as center of tireless service and devotion to others. Women's subordination originated at home and tends to be perpetuated there. Their traditional roles must be revised if women are to be liberated within and through their domestic milieus.

Awareness and realization of identity and commitments may begin at home. By having a place to call their own, women can reflect more effectively about their lives. Women empower themselves through interacting with their families differently rather than by leaving or cutting themselves off from their families, or by meeting all family demands and expectations.

Some of the choices women have about going home are suggested here.

1   Women will only be able to develop their own potential when they honor the importance of being strong. Thus they must transform home into a source of well-being and acknowledge that their fulfillment is a necessity not a luxury.

2   Because consolidation of energies is essential to women's well-being, this goal must be a priority for women if effective change is to occur.

3   Making wholeness their goal rather than perpetuating compartmentalization gives women direction and purpose in their lives.

4   Going home provides a way to recharge and redirect energies. Without regular withdrawal from activity in the outside world, women lose identity and become others' pawns.

5   Going home fosters a new view of oneself. It creates an opportunity for women to revise their identity and commitments. Retreat is necessary for advancement. The pendulum swing of external and internal activities needs to be kept in balance if women are to function effectively and act according to their own interests.

6   Going home for reflection daily increases the effectiveness of women's empowerment.

7   Women take charge of their lives by carving out their own niche at home. Their most meaningful and effective activity derives from contemplation within a self-defined territory.

8   Repeated reflection at home brings about women's metamorphoses. Repetition sustains clarifications of identity and commitments.

9   Peace among people can influence and become peace in the world. Family research suggests that women are more aware of the conditions necessary for peaceful coexistence than are men. Their political contributions in this sphere are crucial for the survival of civilization.

10   Enthusiasm for living is generated by going home to recuperate from daily activities. Going home becomes an integral part of women's lives when they prefer fulfillment to existence.

# Chapter 15

# Fulfillment

It is wholly and uniquely human to ask what the purpose of life is. Fulfillment is personal and social, defined by the choice of goals and ideas an individual makes. We experience fulfillment by contributing to society, not by grasping and being aggressive. We achieve and express fulfillment through social norms and shared values, not in purely idiosyncratic ways.

We choose either to allow life to be lived on its own terms, or to restrict our boundaries and receptivity. Satisfaction is achieved through expansive living rather than through constraints, and it is vital that opportunities for its achievement be available to all.

The restrictiveness of their traditional roles has kept women from fulfillment. The limited number of acceptable roles for women has inhibited their opportunities for expansive living. To move beyond subsistence conditions, women need to be liberated from these limitations. When they engage in broader, more meaningful commitments, the quality of their lives is markedly improved.

Current concerns for women are their need to be themselves and to be responsible members of communities. Traditionally, powerful social conditioning has led women to seek fulfillment by responding to others' needs and demands. However, conflict with these standards and related stereotypes can be productive and rewarding when it moves towards increased satisfactions and increased meaning.

Fulfillment results from spontaneous interaction with others, rather than from endless repetitions of rituals and routines. In order to know ourselves and what our fulfillment requires, we must examine our exchanges in the dyads and triads of our lives. Fulfillment cannot be achieved in isolation or with a few others. If we are to be fulfilled we must maintain an openness and objectivity to all.

Women move towards fulfillment by defining their current situations in meaningful ways. They cannot progress effectively to chosen goals unless they know their circumstances. If they misinterpret who they are, they can redefine themselves by identifying with different values and goals.

Value fulfillment represents a major change for most women. Long conditioned to be satisfied with low levels of self-expression, women live closer to survival than fulfillment. The danger inherent in low expectations is that life becomes devoid of meaning. Enthusiasm and vigor are lost, and the general quality of life diminishes. It is only when women raise their sights and look beyond their immediate survival that they begin the process of fulfillment.

Our fulfillment has to be taken seriously if we are to survive on a long-term basis. Though our lives must perforce be lived at the level of immediacy, we must also seek to transcend the present. Tapping into our deeper potential and future possibilities facilitates realignments in our identity values. Fulfillment increases when values at the core of identity are self-consciously selected. Our love of self and of others redoubles when we move towards fulfillment.

## SELF AND UNIVERSE

Historically women have been restricted in their activities. They have often been prevented and always discouraged from making contributions outside the family or neighborhood. Such limited contact has isolated women and prevented their expansive development. Only when relationships are opened to embrace contacts with wider society can women develop their potential more fully and change structures that limit them.

Fulfillment is the cultivation of a sense of connectedness with others. Identification with selected values enables women to transcend the boundaries of their everyday lives, at the same time becoming more integrated with society. To the extent that their values are universal, women express their oneness with humankind through their chosen identity. Comfort and strength come from knowing one is part of the universe.

An awareness of one's uniqueness and one's interdependency cultivates an open, expansive self-concept. Individual responsibility can no longer be defined in purely personal terms or small group milieus. Identity development requires conscious and deliberate efforts to connect oneself with the universe—with infinity. Concepts of God, religion, or the supernatural generate choices and possibilities for transcendence, hence for the expression of universal dimensions of self.

Women's identity begins to reflect the whole rather than merely traditional expectations. Women abandon their narrow worlds, broadening their lives through expansive decisions. Their shift in focus and vision, and their self-conscious selection of values, enables them to deal more effectively with broader social realities as well as the continuing demands of domestic milieus. The process of relating to wider groups, and to social rather than individual issues, empowers women and increases their fulfillment.

Women's satisfaction evolves through increased awareness and acceptance of their connectedness with the universe. Each woman is a unique participant in evolution. Life's challenge is to negotiate the tension between individuality and universality.

Attentiveness to women's universality increases their motivation to transform social structures which historically have kept them subordinate. Women's efforts to improve circumstances for other women are more effective when they draw freely from universal resources. This process allows women to move beyond the confines of their personal family lives. Contact with social ideals and awareness of their universal connection empower women. This living synthesis of the specific and the universal allows women to get beyond survival and reach fulfillment. Women's biography and history intersect, and structural changes occur as women's potential develops.

## PARTICIPATING IN EVOLUTION

Each person participates in evolution. Fulfillment increases through knowing that each of us is an active part of this process. To belong to something bigger than the self is essential to living expansively.

Awareness of being part of evolution suggests some limitations as well as opportunities for women's individual and collective action. One limitation is the realization that quantum leaps in substantive change cannot be produced by random efforts or ordinary circumstances. In the normal course of events the deepest changes occur slowly, generally as a result of very prolonged new patterns of activity.

Opportunities for action can be based on the knowledge of how human potential is developed. Evolution is both a context and a source of explanation for such analysis. For example, research in the physical sciences has shown that the human brain has become larger and more complex during recent

evolutionary stages. This increase, more rapid than other physiological re-
finements, underscores that a greater emphasis on intellectual over physical
strength opens up a wide berth of opportunities for women to contribute to
society.

False parallels between evolution and specific kinds of social change are
misleading. Only broad-brush applications of evolution to society and individuals can be made. One of the most significant extensions of the idea of evolution to human behavior, and to women's behavior in particular, is that the
human body is a delicate instrument which has extraordinary powers. Although
we cannot fully assess or understand our bodies, we know that our human
faculties have increased in recent phases of evolution. Current research on
"right brain" behavior, for example, suggests that what we have traditionally
defined as women's intuition is a strong creative impulse, a constructive power.
Women's energies and capacities can be directed to society more effectively
when their real interests and goals are identified.

Survival necessitates access to collective resources and group protection.
Women need other women in order to survive. Only the collective action of
women can, in the long run, accomplish the structuring of equal opportunities
for all women. Women are fulfilled when they orient their energies towards
improving the life conditions of other women. Whereas their efforts to survive
as individuals are ultimately destructive, their awareness that they are connected with other women enhances their experience and moves them towards
fulfillment.

Evolutionary dynamics are believed to create increasingly complex nuances
in human behavior and the human condition. Cognitive and psychic phenomena
may be more important in human communication and functioning than previously supposed. Women's trust in the forces of the universe within and outside
them heightens their sense of being. Religious faith may also be strengthened
by evolutionary awareness, largely through a sense of universal connections.
Although human powerlessness may be accentuated by considering evolution,
our willingness to surrender to life processes can be increased.

Women's knowledge of evolution promotes their acceptance of life as a
moving force working through them. While passivity inhibits life, women's
liberation and fulfillment opens them to the flow of life across time and space.

## EMPOWERMENT

Empowerment is a strengthening of individuals and groups which occurs
through interaction at all levels of social organization. Empowerment begins
with identity clarification and includes the making of commitments for action in
society. Empowerment processes are constructive and not destructive. They
enhance purpose and cause in individuals' and groups' motivation. Evolutionary processes move towards increasing empowerment. Empowerment is en-

hanced by women's awareness of their participation in evolution. Empowerment results from seeing and knowing connections between now and eternity, the finite and infinite.

Empowerment results from imbuing activity with meaning, and the process itself generates meaning. The deliberate selection of our values deepens our bonds to life and allows us to interact with others more effectively. Empowerment enables us to transcend circumstances by putting us in touch with our own immortality. In transcending the present, we broaden our perspectives and horizons to include timeless dimensions of existence. Detachment increases our objectivity, a vital component of empowerment.

Women's lives flow more easily and have a broader scope when they are empowered. Strengthening identity is an escape from entrapment, which allows women to have a meaningful point of departure for their participation in the world.

Empowerment provides more equal conditions than empirical realities generally allow. It enables women to look at the world more freely and to decide what it is they can change in their current life circumstances.

Empowerment is a means for women to assess where they are and what they would like to do. This consolidation of energies and resources is increased through women's collective action. Together they accomplish more than individual women can, however exceptional and talented an individual woman may be.

Women are their own source of motivation. Their cause of equality cannot be satisfactorily achieved until equal opportunities for all are established and maintained. Women can be a clearly defined and effective force in society and the transformation of social structures.

Women's new power is generated by their transition from passivity to activity, from limited perspectives to broad horizons. This process puts women in touch with their own needs and real interests, enabling them to be strengthened through contacts with other women. Their increased trust in self and others enables women to break out of limiting isolation. Intuitive leads enhance their empowerment and ultimate fulfillment.

Empowerment is growth and development and defines possibilities and goals for women. Women gain in substance and power when they move away from the traditional and historical restrictions that have demanded fragility and passivity from them. Diverse kinds of power are embraced by women as they clarify their choices in identity, being, and activity.

## WOMEN'S FULFILLMENT

Women's fulfillment is similar to that of men. However, historically women's definitions of reality have differed significantly from men's. While men have concerned themselves with economic and political realities, women have seen their lives through family and religious definitions. Both women and men need to develop their potential. Human liberation and full participation are shared goals, and balanced relations between women and men can only develop through cooperative partnership.

Historically women's isolation and restrictions have alienated them more than men. Identity and value choices are crucial aspects of women's fulfillment. They must define clearly who they are and where they want to go before they can begin to move out of their subordination. In this process women's differences from men must be acknowledged, and their perceptions and definitions of reality endorsed.

Many similarities between women and men exist—similarities that must not be obscured by overemphasis on gender distinctiveness. With overlapping sensibilities and talents, both women and men aspire to have satisfying lives. Women are beginning to realize their strengths are comparable to men's. Women can be fulfilled by developing what are considered to be "male" identity assets, just as men can be fulfilled by developing sensitivities and sensibilities conventionally ascribed to females. Women and men are whole persons, all having the broadest range of human characteristics.

Women's fulfillment necessitates broadening the scope of their activities and enlarging their worlds. Men, on the other hand may need to slow down or restrict their lives, in order to become more directly influenced by their inner promptings.

Women must not form their own elites since this would lead to the exclusion of some women and the partial fulfillment of others. They can benefit only from equal opportunities for all. Furthermore, the fulfillment of women and men must coexist. Alienation prevents the achievement of real equality and full participation.

Currently, both women and men pay too high a price for their life choices. Their activities frequently do not reflect real needs or interests. Men appear to be fulfilled. They have generally achieved this at the expense of others, however, particularly of women and men with the fewest resources. Exploitation and oppression bring penalties for all. Only equality in personal and public relations can be in everyone's best interest.

Women must believe in the possibility of fulfillment before they can be fulfilled. In order to survive in the long run, fulfillment must be real for women. Women transcend their harsh empirical realities, as well as survival levels of behavior, by planning and undertaking activities which move them towards fulfillment.

The development of women's and men's potential requires action in directions of fulfillment. Living the good life must be for all—people cannot benefit in the long run from impinging on the freedom of others.

## COMPLETION

Fulfillment is a satisfying sense of completion. Although accustomed to thinking about time as unilinear, we should more productively view our lives as comprised of different stages, rhythms, and cycles. The varied responsibilities women assume throughout a lifetime, particularly in modern industrial societies, are patterned by their roles. Women may seem to live many different lives within the chronology of a single lifetime, as the nature of these roles may change dramatically.

Completion requires that we selectively include or exclude specific activities in our daily routines. We need to look at what it is that would bring wholeness and completion to our values and commitments. Identity concerns motivate us to discover what would make us complete as individuals.

In order to be fulfilled, it is necessary to make our action complete. Thus, we must surrender ourselves to our best impulses and seek total self-acceptance. We must consider all women in understanding our experiences and in defining our responsibilities. We can only become effective and fulfilled agents of change by complete commitment to the cause of equality for all. Our most complete act may be living as an equal, as a full partner, and as a full participant in evolution.

This means that we participate in preparing the world for our children and our children's children. We cannot accomplish everything we would like to in our own lifetimes, but we can move towards establishing more equal conditions for all.

We gain peace of mind when we become fully immersed in our efforts to achieve that which we value most. Belief in equality is belief in life itself. When we value the uniqueness and independence of each person as fully as we do our own, we encourage strong and cooperative relationships. Equality becomes a foundation for greater human productivity and finer accomplishment.

It is only be bestowing a quality of sacredness on equality that society will be enhanced. If society is to flourish, equality has to be our highest priority and primary concern. In order to have meaning in our lives, we must make a full commitment to the goal of equality. Partial commitment is too easily neutralized. We are empowered when we are completely invested in our identity as an equal.

This degree of totality of effort brings time into focus and orients us towards giving to others. Being here in the present allows us to synthesize the past and future. We touch eternity.

Fulfillment requires complete effort and results from contributing to others' well-being. We give of ourselves most fully when we have self-knowledge and committed identity. Equality establishes structures, processes, and states of mind. We are only free to be ourselves when we are equal.

## PERFECTION

As an almost imperceptible dimension of reality, perfection appears to elude human endeavor. When we start with the assumption that there is as yet undiscovered perfect peace and harmony in the universe, we can find excellence in our experience.

As a belief or an ideology, perfection is an effective means of moving people towards improved social conditions. Ideals in human conduct and in social relationships are articulated by most religious belief systems. The concept of God is a social or human expression of perfection and perfect process.

Perfection embraces harmonies which may appear to be disharmonies. Conflict is appropriate and valuable when it moves us towards constructive change. Conflict is also a stage of healing that culminates in wholeness and perfection.

Conscious identity allows women to see and appreciate their own uniqueness and genius. The expression of women's genius is one kind of newfound perfection of being. Women's shift from oppression to valuing and articulating their genius is a revolution.

Acknowledging that perfection already exists requires us to examine our lives and living conditions closely. In contemplation and meditation we become deliberately inactive, waiting to be enlightened or moved by powers beyond ourselves. Women can cultivate attitudes of awe and enchantment which generate spontaneity beyond the direct influence of thought and emotional control. We become ourselves in a stream of perfection.

Women's equality with men is both a means and an end. We catch a glimpse of perfection only when we allow each other to be ourselves. Equality, then, gives direction to our expression of a perfection that already exists.

Equality allows us to know and realize perfection. When we acknowledge equality in our thoughts, feelings, and deeds, we are more fulfilled and better able to achieve excellence. Order and harmony may not be easily discerned, but equality underlies and permeates our essence and existence.

This utopian analysis of women's and men's equality engenders ideals and beliefs that have practical consequences for thoughts, perceptions, values, and solutions. We are less entangled in the structures of our lives than caught in discordant value and belief systems. When we clarify and revise our values, and value our identity, we get out of many of the traps that have been created. Until they see reality for what it is, and value their own uniqueness as well as their shared strengths, women and men remain enemies. Empowerment springs from belief in perfection and possibilities, and from individual and collective efforts to be honest and open in thinking and action.

## GENERALIZATIONS AND PROPOSITIONS

Fulfillment suggests deliberate action in response to human realities. Passivity brings frustration and entrapment, not fulfillment. By acknowledging that there are practical ways to move towards fulfillment, we understand and achieve human possibilities more fully.

Generalizations about orienting women's actions towards increased fulfillment follow.

1  Whatever their circumstances, fulfillment is possible for all women and all people.

2  Fulfillment is experienced and expressed in a multitude of diverse ways relating to individual values and circumstances.

3  In fulfillment women transcend their private experiences to an awareness of their connectedness with the universe and human evolution.

4  The satisfaction and empowerment that fulfillment brings urges us toward a perfection that exists with or without us.

5  Women's fulfillment is similar to men's; both require equal access to resources, opportunities, and rewards.

6  Fulfillment brings with it a sense of completion—that one is doing what one is meant to do.

7  Fulfillment is necessary for long-run survival.

More specific propositions about fulfillment can also be formulated.

1  Women cannot be fulfilled at the expense of men, nor can men be fulfilled at the cost of women's oppression.

2  Women must rise above creating elites in their being and behavior—only equality can bring the freedom both women and men need.

3  Currently it is women, not men, who take the initiative to achieve fulfillment, but ultimately all humans will be included.

4  Women's fulfillment derives from expressions of their genius and excellence in all activity.

5  Women's fulfillment is an essential part of a harmonious reality brought into being through value changes.

6  Fulfillment is a prerequisite for all humans, not a luxury for the privileged few. When we deliberately work towards our fulfillment, we participate in our own evolution.

7  Fulfillment is both completion and beginning; it is a vantage point from which to evaluate our lives and the life of our society.

Chapter 16

# Conclusion

We live in a dazzling world that offers many options. It is difficult to establish priorities among these choices. Guidelines are essential if we are to honor life and contribute to others to our fullest capacity.

Our identity is the source of our thinking, feeling, and acting. We discover ourselves and choose to change ourselves. Our commitments and behavior flow directly from our identity. Identity is both impersonal or objective and subjective. We are linked to others through our identity, and through the values we cherish. Identity defines our uniqueness and at the same time pulls us into social integration. We become unified with others through selected ideals that transcend the subjective or limited self. Identity broadens our base of belonging with others and includes a sense of belonging with the whole of humankind. Women become aware of their womanhood within the context of the human race and the human condition.

Emphasis on the significance of identity implies that our choices in this changing world are not of equal importance and do not have comparable consequences. Diverse consequences develop from both a close examination of identity and deliberate choices of identity. Activities of identity discernment and identity construction have a greater influence on our lives than other goals and commitments.

Identity concerns are particularly significant for women. Throughout history women have been discouraged from knowing and meeting their own needs and from delineating their own interests. They have been preoccupied with sustenance and maintenance tasks without the opportunity to consider their place in the total scheme of things. During the 20th century, however, increasing numbers of women have begun to examine women's concerns in their own terms. This increased awareness facilitates identity empowerment and enhances their lives.

Women's freedom is significantly increased by changes in legislation and changes in men's behavior. Identity clarification includes working for these particular improvements. Engagement of women's spirit is more essential to equal rights, however, as this encourages and motivates women to claim the good life as their entitlement. Men are not motivated to do this for women! We are finite beings who have a moral responsibility to designate our time and energy for particular purposes. Present efforts to understand and create identity pay rich dividends. Women progress towards a more tolerant and humane community by being autonomous, by not reacting to the expectations of others. Identity empowerment brings women into balanced relations with men. It increases their participation and the effectiveness of their contributions to society's power and authority structures. Our mutual long-range survival depends on the ability of women and men to select life-enhancing values—such as equality, love, and truth—as sources of identity.

Theoretically, the need to focus on identity and initiate value changes in society is as much in the interest of men as of women. However, as only women are consistently subordinated in society, their need to empower identity is more acute then men's. Women's pain and despair become impetus and opportunity for their growth and increased expansiveness in living.

## ENLIGHTENMENT

Women are in the midst of their own social movement, which is propelled by new and different ideas. The modern feminist enlightenment emphasizes the same freedom and reason that characterizes the European enlightenment of the 18th and 19th centuries. Current changes also center on equality, but this time equality is expressed through the feminine values of nurturing care, support for life, peace, and harmony.

Egalitarian forms of community replace hierarchical forms. Feminism moves us out of the dark ages of ignorance and oppression. Everyone becomes able to recognize their real needs and to see their lives in broader perspective. Education removes some of the restrictions that held women captive in repetitions of traditional behavior. As well as choosing different roles, women more knowledgeably reflect about all their roles, and make more deliberate choices about the direction of their lives.

Women live fully as soon as they claim equality for themselves. They cannot afford to wait for laws to bring equality to them, even though the legislative protection of women's equality is necessary and vital to women's well-being. In the meantime, women must empower themselves by acknowledging and accepting their equal worth as human beings.

Enlightenment is a realization that there are many choices to make. We choose how we think and what we do, and eventually what we feel. Our thoughts influence how we feel, especially when we select our most important values and goals as our highest priorities. This is a necessary condition for realizing our potential, and for connecting with religions or belief systems of our choice. We realize possibilities, call forth life, move forward, and do something worthwhile.

We are enlightened when we see our lives for what they are rather than as others have defined them. We transcend empirical difficulties and complexities, and burdens are discarded. When identity is a central concern, we realize that we are life itself. Our freedom enhances our reason. We become more in charge of our lives and less at the mercy of others. We discern objectives that are in our own interest and select effective means to move towards them. We give what we can to others and respect their talents and freedom.

Women's transformation can be empirically substantiated. Clinical data show that we cannot return to living as we did before without physiological or social penalties. We are in individual and social metamorphosis. Women's thinking and behavior transforms them and society.

Women's heightened awareness is a means to an end, not their goal. Their progress culminates in their continuing contribution to society. Women enhance life and strengthen constructive life forces through their clear thinking, decision-making, and behavior.

The crux of these changes is equality. Women who identify with the value of equality live as equals. Deliberate identification is necessary to neutralize the flow of convention and conformity that pushes women forcefully into traditional subordinate positions. Women are victims of institutionalized inequalities and only women's active claims of equal worth can bring equality into being.

Enlightenment is seeing the priority of priorities. Women order their lives through empowered action when they accept reality and themselves. Restrictions become alien and dissolve, and they live fully.

## HISTORY

History is not a fixed record and facts cannot speak for themselves. In order to reflect the complexity of society and change, history needs to be revised and rewritten from a variety of perspectives. No single person or class of people can give a sufficiently full and deep account of events through time.

Women's history has not yet been written, although feminist scholars currently contribute many new kinds of knowledge through their research. Assumptions about reality and human nature are challenged by new data about women and women's interpretations of facts. Cross-cultural studies are another significant source of new knowledge about women.

Identity concerns and value choices increase women's opportunities to become significant historical actors. They become better able to change institutionalized patterns of behavior by becoming aware of broad change processes. History demands our participation if we intend that our actions have a significant impact on society. Women ignore this call for participation when they merely react to the push and pull of others' pressures and expectations. Clinical data show that it is easier to be submerged by history than to be an actor in change processes.

Recorded history is unkind and unjust to women. Women's achievements have been ignored or at best sketchily documented. Women who internalize male values and accept limited leadership roles in male patriarchies are honored more than women who are anonymous laborers in female subcultures. Few histories of women's restricted domestic milieus or histories of lower-class women have been written and accepted as knowledge.

Women work towards equality when they increase their historical awareness. The history of social thought traces the idea and ideal of equality to Greek and Roman Stoic philosophy, as well as to early Christian communities. The ideal of equality was lost in the dark ages of medieval feudalism, and did not reemerge until the 18th and 19th century age of reason and enlightenment in Europe.

Today the ideal of equality has new significance. The feminist enlightenment of the 20th century emphasizes different aspects of equality, and survival and fulfillment functions of equal partnership between women and men are more urgent.

We cannot ignore or deny history—we decide to act on its challenge. We are historic beings through language and circumstance. Women's passive acceptance of others' power is no more an inevitable outcome than their leadership and active participation in change. However, women direct the course of history only when they have historical awareness and realize preferred options though decisions and deliberate action.

Women's quest for identity strengthens their autonomy and power. Historical reviews of events in women's lives show patterns in their value commitments. This review can also be usefully extended to include women's activities in several generations of family histories. The broader the historical perspective women can take on their own behavior, the more objective they can be in their assessment of their own autonomy. When women see how the women emotionally closest to them live, they are better able to see their own lives in perspective and more likely to place a higher value on their own lives.

When they are informed about past centuries of women's history, women are united in their efforts to achieve equality. Through historical research, well-founded appeals and claims to the moral ideal of justice are made. To be full participants and contributors to the common good, women need equality before the law and equality in moral worth. Women have innate equality and worth which must be honored in all social negotiations.

Language and values anchor us in history. We cannot escape the effects of our Judeo–Christian heritage. We respond to this heritage most appropriately and most freely through understanding the history of these traditions. Women also deepen their understanding of their heritage by comparing and contrasting Western values with traditional Eastern belief systems. An in-depth examination of historic religions shows that not all religious values restrict women's lives. Religious beliefs that deepen their understanding of life support women as they deal with historical realities. Religious beliefs also help women to transcend historical realities of the present, bringing them to new, more rewarding levels of existence. History reminds us about our past, but does not define all our options. We need history to give us direction and purpose, and to enable us to transcend the present and build a more fulfilling future.

## DREAMS

Utopian vision generates change. Consciously created dreams in the realm of possibility give a sense of direction and purpose to planned activity and behavior. Women need dreams which carry them forward.

Dreams are not always fortuitous products of the subconscious. Dreams may be deliberately constructed and used as goals for social action. Dreams are at the heart of political activism.

Women's challenge of the present is to create new forms of social structure. Equality is the central value of the feminist enlightenment, and a primary ideal for the invention of new social forms. When dreams are founded upon a principle of equality, they continue civilizations of the past and create a different future.

Change is cultivated when priorities are organized around the ideal of equality. Planning for a community of equals transforms traditional patterns of interaction. Although Judeo–Christian religions are not completely based upon acceptance of unequal relationships, inequality has been a powerful value in Judeo–Christian patriarchies of the West. Equal worth has existed only as an unattainable ideal.

In contrast to dreams, fantasy is an escape from reality. In fantasy, images are entertained purposely to transport people from their present circumstances into an unreal world. Dreams, especially deliberately constructed daydreams, are mechanisms that deal with reality. Specific plans evolve from dreams, showing us how to move towards them.

Dreams develop in the minds of individuals, but are easily shared. A collective dream establishes bonds between people and galvanizes them into action. Women's identity can be a dream or ideal at individual and collective levels. As women share their dream of equality, they move towards real equality. Dreaming is action and not passive reaction. Dreams direct activities to goals.

Dreams activate the imagination. We imagine the implications of ideals in order to know what we want most. Women have tended to imagine negative rather than positive outcomes of their restricted lives. However, they can move into life's expansiveness by deliberately dreaming about solutions to restrictions, not by contemplating the many aspects of their limitations.

Dangers of dreaming lurk in the zone between fantasizing and dreaming. Although fantasy serves a useful function as release for both the oppressed and unoppressed, fantasy's unreal quality makes it impractical or counterproductive in everyday life. Women have to know where they are and what they want so that their hopes can become realistic dreams and plans for action.

By associating identity and value choices, women dream their way out of traditional restrictions. Women's discernment of values that liberate them generates dreams that provide adaptations to traditions. This process is not so much thinking our way out of problems, as deciding to imagine and create solutions.

Dreams bypass intolerable realities. They guide us from past to future. Women become historical actors by first seeing themselves as historical actors. We rise to meet the needs of situations we find ourselves in by seeing our action through dreams.

Thus, dreams are our beginning and end. We see what has to be done before we can do it. The feminist enlightenment is a substitution of viable dreams for unpleasant and damaging realities. Our dreams also build a history in that we create history now for the future. Dreams are the heart of political activism and liberation. Although the dreams of women and men may be different, we all need dreams for survival and fulfillment.

## FUTURES

Part of the challenge of being a woman in contemporary society is that women's lives are increasingly unpredictable. Not only do women carve out lives that are distinct from those of their mothers and grandmothers, but they also live different stages of their lives in dramatically different ways. Women's futures are unclear, but increased freedom rather than restriction characterizes this lack of predictability. Women are more able to design their future than before, despite the fact that institutionalized gender inequalities continue to limit their possibilities.

Social and political activism become more effective when they are directed towards the future. Strategies immersed in the past or programs geared towards short-term solutions do not have as lasting impacts on society as action oriented towards long-range change. Women's hopes are inevitably tilted towards the future as their past is imbued with despair. Women do the most they can in the present by using the past as a starting point, mapping out constructive conditions for a more satisfying future in the present.

Women create futures that evolve from choices they make now. Belief in the primary importance of equality transforms the nature of relationships at all levels of society, and ultimately transforms society itself. As women translate their central belief in equality into action, they build families and communities which have new structures. These new forms of family and community neutralize the formidable power of institutionalized patriarchal inequalities. The principle of equal worth enables us to accept all simultaneously, with deepened understanding and support for their growth and development as human beings.

Orientation to a specific future compels us to formulate goals. Consideration of a world outside women's domestic milieus necessitates the definition of objectives which affect others. The more women turn their skills in nurturing care to the well-being of society as a whole, the more they are fulfilled through their deliberate actions. They find themselves when they discover what they are most able to give to others.

Historical perspectives enable women to identify with one another and with the flow of history itself. Women's awareness of historical dimensions of the social movement of feminism makes them actors rather than reactors to the currents of change. They may choose to work toward the transcendence of gender in the future, but for the moment they need to specify their oneness with all women's values. When women know their heritage of subordination under patriarchalism, they launch themselves more effectively into a freedom of reason, liberty, and equality. Ideals become realities in women's lives as they move towards a changed future through deliberate choices in values and act with integrity for liberated identity. The mere formulation of opinion and action prompted by whim are inadequate. Women must take principled stands, and act according to belief in an underlying reality of equal worth with others in all their thoughts, attitudes, and behavior.

The feminist enlightenment, at both personal and collective levels, shows us how women learn from one another and build a more life-enhancing future. This experience crosses all social classes and all cultures. Women and men are united by their common heritage of the human condition, and by their mutual desires and intentions to improve the quality of life for all. Women's circles of contacts with each other become ever more inclusive through time. They are at peace only when there is well-being for all.

Today, women's ideas influence history more directly than before. Their primary value of equal worth brings balance to all levels of social structure and interaction. Feminist consciousness heals social ills in modern society.

Our futures are created now. Time is not a simple, linear phenomenon. Our connections with the past breathe life into the future through the facts of our present existence. The strength of women's orientation to life enhances the possibility that their future will be better than today. The feminist challenge transforms existing limitations to freer realities for women and men.


## CHALLENGE

Each woman and man is challenged to assess who they are and where they are going. Women's two main options are to accept this challenge positively and reorder their lives or suppress the challenge and suffer. Both women and men harm themselves by any inability to define their being as source of action and values.

The feminist challenge labels us as creatures of equal worth in the human condition. Our world appears different from the egalitarian perspective that we are no more and no less than others. Women must decide to treat themselves as equals and refuse to carry on the patriarchal tradition of limiting or sacrificing themselves for others.

The feminist challenge makes women question their conditioned behavior. They can no longer survive by putting their lives on automatic pilot and hoping for the best. Enlightenment is an awakening to the challenge of being a woman.

The most supreme value choice women make is an assessment of who they are. A person's sense of worth and power derive from this assessment. Do human beings have limited or unlimited potential? Can personal or individual power influence patriarchal structures? Can a woman rebel effectively against others' expectations, and thrive without harming herself? Can women afford to challenge and change patriarchal values?

Women build a future that embodies feminist values if they believe they are of equal worth and their values are significant. They must become agents of change if their children are to survive and be fulfilled, and they must assume their responsibilities as full participants in society if institutions are to become balanced. By thinking inclusively women carve out freedom from the restrictions of their domestic milieus.

The feminist enlightenment allows women to transcend many of the limits of their historical context. They recognize that it is possible for them to reach other women and men in order to build new community structures and new worlds. Universalism is part of the vision of the feminist enlightenment. Women's struggle for life is the struggle of every woman, and there can be no rest for women until they have improved the lot of all women.

The feminist enlightenment reveals the importance of choices. Each moment brings with it possibilities for decisions that have individual and social consequences. Women need to be fully alert to know what their best interests are and how their action affects others. They come out of the shadows of patriarchy into the light of egalitarianism.

The feminist challenge touches the depths of women's souls—their love, aspirations, and loyalties. Although women's reaction may be to withdraw from this challenge once they have seen the possibilities, they cannot retreat. Women's vision compels them to move forward and make progress. Their lives are channeled in new directions.

When heart and soul accept self, and endorse commitment to the feminist challenge, women's plans blossom and their actions bear fruit. Development of potential depends on their whole-hearted embrace of the invitation to contribute women's values to society. Rejection of this opportunity inevitably has negative consequences for all.

Challenge manifests in women's external affairs and within them. They feel discomfort in the old ways of doing things. It is such uneasiness that spurs their curiosity and heightens their need to define themselves in ways that will meet the challenge. If they sink back into patriarchy, they lose themselves. They realize this with joy, relief, and heartbreak. Can women risk giving up the familiar in order to move into the unknown?

Women are empowered to choose enlightenment by knowing that this is a personal responsibility. They gain mutual support through friendship with women. Their enlightenment is an ongoing collective effort, and each woman loses her fears in their shared trust, faith, and confidence. This challenge is for us all, and no one needs to face choices alone. We grow through connections of effort, and creative community replaces destructive power.

## GENERALIZATIONS AND PROPOSITIONS

These generalizations and propositions derive from many hundreds of life histories of women who are changing the quality of their lives through value choices. Although the significance of identity and value choices in women's lives has not yet been definitively documented, exploratory research and observation show that this process plays a crucial role in women's empowerment. Women can change their social positions and they can work toward changing social structures to free themselves and others.

No distillation of the complex detail of life histories is fully representative. Summations and emphases omit important parts of the real picture. However, a charting of repeated patterns of behavior is helpful in formulating a direction in which to work or a goal for which to strive.

Several important generalizations about women and identity are listed below.

1   Women recognize social influences that restrict them and values which orient them to more expansive living.
2   Goals of fulfillment are more satisfying to women than survival objectives.

**3**  When women know they are equals, they live as equals.

**4**  By identifying themselves with life in the universe, women are motivated to transcend personal limitations.

**5**  Women's identity is the stimulus for action that changes the patriarchal structures that limit women's growth and fulfillment.

**6**  Women help other women to see who they are through friendship and support.

**7**  Women's identity is historical, and they become actors by taking advantage of opportunities for change.

More specific propositions flow from these generalizations and highlight the kinds of actual choices women make as they live more fully. When women more accurately define their situation, they are able to choose their direction more precisely. These generalizations and propositions rest on the assumption that women and men are of equal worth.

The following propositions address the significance of identity for women.

**1**  The more aware women are of the deepest roots of their identity, the more effective they will be as historical actors.

**2**  Women's identity is defined most clearly by examining their roles in family, work, community, and friendships.

**3**  Religion is a powerful influence on identity, and the more women's values endorse their freedom, the freer they will be.

**4**  To the extent that identity is linked with mission or purpose, women are more likely to be fulfilled. Religion or spirituality are guides for women's long-range action.

**5**  Increasing women's understanding of family relationships gives them more freedom from family pressures and expectations. Families are a significant site of oppression for women; thus commitment to examine family histories is an important mechanism of change.

**6**  Women's identity relates to empirical realities, and at the same time transcends them. When women see the possibilities for change, they are more likely to rise out of difficult situations.

**7**  The most important commitment women make to enhance their life satisfaction is to maintain efforts to increase their awareness of identity and its implied goals.

## CHOICES

Women have vital choices to make. Though they cannot select conditions in their environment, they can choose values that define identity and meaning in their lives. However disastrous a particular situation may appear to be, women have choices, if only the basic choice of how to be in the universe they experience. Women's choices (especially those made thoughtfully) promote changes that ultimately enhance life for all.

Choices are unique and respond to particular situations. There are principles which define bases for women's decision-making. The following choices address issues which relate to women's selection of values for identity formation and the expression of identity through action.

**1** The value of equality is central to the real interests of women. Valuing equality as primary in all settings enables women to see themselves differently, and it inspires new modes of activity.

**2** Choices exist at every moment of existence. When women increase the deliberateness of their choices, they become correspondingly more responsible for the consequences of their action.

**3** Women choose to empower their sense of who they are by selecting powerful values as foundation for their being and activity. Life, love, truth, freedom, and equality are traditional values women choose that improve their functioning in the world.

**4** By choosing action over passivity, women transform their lives and deal with circumstances more effectively.

**5** Women choose to empower themselves by valuing their friendships and exchanges with other women. Mutual support among women is essential to consolidate their resources and modify restrictive structures.

**6** Women choose inclusive values. Their communities do not exclude men, but rather create different patterns of equal exchanges and mutual support in full partnerships with men.

**7** Women's choice of equality creates symmetrical, harmonious family structures. Intimate relationships become more autonomous and freer in their interdependency.

**8** Women choose to attain the good life for themselves without impinging on the rights or freedom of others. Women realize their increased satisfaction through availing themselves of the multiple opportunities that present themselves.

**9** Women choose to trust others, and to have faith in the constructive, intelligent life forces in the universe. By accepting the challenge of living positively, women affirm their strength through action.

**10** Women choose to place a priority on maintaining their identity awareness. Other choices and commitments flow from their basic self-definition. When women know who they are, they know where to go!

# Clinical Sociology

*Women and Identity* is based on a particular clinical sociological theory. Life-history data collected in both clinical and research settings are sources used for the development of the concepts presented (Thomas, 1927). Identity empowerment describes a personal and social strengthening process which is used as a tool by clinical sociologists and therapists to improve the quality of life and living conditions of clients. The optimal outcome of therapeutic intervention is a continuing, high degree of identity empowerment in personal and social settings.

Clinical sociology is a frame of reference and substantive discipline that generates many effective change strategies for practitioners and clients (Glassner & Freedman, 1979; Lee, 1955; Straus, 1979; Swan, 1984; Wirth, 1931). The interdependent concepts in clinical sociological theory provide a new view of individual and social functioning. As a body of substantive knowledge, clinical sociology describes and seeks to explain the influence of both broad and narrow social structures on interpersonal behavior (Gerth & Mills, 1953; Mead, 1934; Mills, 1959). The discipline of clinical sociology suggests the following propositions.

1   Personal problems must be deliberately related to contexts of immediate and broad social structures in order to gain objectivity and achieve a more accurate understanding of the influence of milieus on individual behavior.

2   A redefinition of personal problems generates an increased number of choices for participants in the settings examined (Straus, 1984).

3   Conflict resolution is essentially a learning process. Clinicians help their clients to observe and understand their experiences more fully. Information gathered about patterns in conflicts is used for precipitating further change.

Life-history data reveal great diversity in patterns of decision-making throughout life courses. Major events are crucial turning points that significantly influence decision-making processes.

Values and relationships are reforged in times of crisis, and individuals or groups may lose their effectiveness and become dysfunctional. Therapeutic intervention in crises strengthens capacities to adapt or change. Identity empowerment is one of the most advantageous outcomes of therapeutic intervention. Identity empowerment is increased autonomy and increased awareness of choices leading ultimately to revised commitments with broad social consequences. Identity empowerment occurs when new views of self and the universe are formulated and their related values incorporated in daily living.

Crisis intervention by clinical sociologists increases the probability that these turning points are perceived as opportunities for learning and change by clients, thereby having constructive outcomes (Garfinkel, 1967). Changes in the behavior of individuals also modify social structures. To the extent that individuals' awareness is increased, they will assume leadership or more influential positions in old and new groups, facilitating structural changes as a consequence of the shifts in their own levels of activity and commitment.

Health can be thought of as experiences of well-being for individuals, and effective goal-oriented activities for both individuals and groups. The main focus of interest in clinical observations and theory construction is examining, encouraging, and achieving behavior which falls within a range of health and effective functioning.

Data collected and used as sources for conceptualization in this book are individual and family life histories rather than larger group histories. Discussions in *Women and Identity* center on applications of clinical sociology concepts to women. These concepts are sometimes applied to relationships between larger groups as well as to interaction.

Ten concepts are used to develop effective strategies from this clinical sociological theory. Social interaction is conceptualized as the negotiation of values (Berger & Luckman, 1966; Blumer, 1969; Cooley, 1964; Goffman, 1959; Homans, 1961), and all people are thought of as negotiating values with each other. Identity empowerment results from strengthening clients' capacities through more conscious, deliberate value choices in their lives. The ranges of values considered as baselines for interpersonal and intergroup negotiations, choices, and commitments include material and nonmaterial values as well as traditional and modern values.

## CONCEPTUAL SCHEMA

Each of the 10 concepts used is described briefly in order to present a holistic view of interrelationships among them. The sequence of concepts below represents a continuously increasing span of substantive concerns, from micro to macro relationships of individuals and social structures. The animating dynamics in these processes are conceptualized as negotiations of values. Negotiations may not have compatible outcomes because value differences may disrupt interaction.

Identity empowerment is built upon awareness of the extent to which micro and macro structures influence the quality of personal and public life. This understanding results in an enhanced capacity to take value stands on personal and public issues. When deepened understanding and broadened perspectives come into play with identity processes, constructive values are deliberately selected through more aware decision-making. Clinical sociology applications in therapeutic crisis intervention work toward the identity empowerment of clients.

Ten basic concepts of this clinical sociological theory follow.

### 1. Self

*Self* is the conceptualization of who we are in relation to others. No substantial increase in functioning effectiveness can occur without a person's continuous scrutiny of patterns of interaction, especially with significant others. Personal character is directly related to micro and macro structures in that milieus have a direct influence on behavior. It is generally too difficult for most people to see and understand this connectedness. Both negotiable and nonnegotiable values are the product of socialization and resocialization.

### 2. Dyad

A *dyad* is a two-person or two-group relationship which is characterized by subordination and superordination interaction patterns. A preliminary step towards seeing oneself in a context of social structures at different levels of organization is to examine the variety of "routinized" dyads in which an individual participates. Patterns of dominance or submissiveness are delineated, and degrees of stress and precariousness noted. Symbiosis, or extreme mutual dependence, and less dramatic forms of dependency are also delineated in this process of observing and examining significant dyads.

### 3. Triad

A *triad* is a three-person or three-group relationship that generally has two insiders and one outsider. A triad is the most stable micro structure that exists (Caplow, 1968; Simmel, 1950). If one person leaves a triad, the remaining dyad pulls a substitute third party into their relationship, thus perpetuating the triad. When a dyad has high levels of anxiety or stress, it is predictable that a third party will be drawn into the twosome.

The most intense emotional involvement between two people in a triad can be positively close or conflictual. The third person is outside the emotional field of dyadic closeness or conflict. The outsider position is generally not preferred when the other two people are emotionally close, but it is preferred when they are in conflict. In all instances the outsider position is strongest because this functioning position is the most autonomous. Although no triad stays balanced for long periods of time, through the equal participation of all three persons, the outsider position continues to be less restricted than the two insider positions which are caught up in the intense dependency of closeness or conflict.

### 4. Family

*Family* may be thought of as a metaphor representing a person's most meaningful relationships as well as a concept that implies position and functioning in a group based on kinship or contract. A family is a relatively open relationship system encompassing members of several generations. Family is the most intensely dependent group to which an individual belongs.

### 5. Religion

*Religion* is used here as a metaphor to describe a person's beliefs about visible and invisible realities. Everyday beliefs or organized, traditional religious beliefs are tied to social structures. Individuals' religions may include combinations of denominational, sectarian, traditional, modern, and secular beliefs. Ways in which we perceive the universe through others' beliefs, or through our own individual chosen beliefs, must be distinguished and examined.

### 6. Definition of the Situation

How we define the different situations of our lives reflects our understanding of self, society, and the universe. We view all physical and social conditions with value perspectives, and define our choices accordingly. Our definitions strongly influence our motivation and help to form our assumptions and goals. Our beliefs about self and reality have social sources and bring critical social consequences, creating parameters of our personal and public behavior (Thomas, 1931).

## 7. Reference Group

The intensity of our sense of belonging to specific groups, and our identification with these groups, has special meaning for us. Our affiliation with chosen reference groups is a strong influence on our behavior. This influence is powerful whether we actually belong to a group or merely aspire to group membership. The values of our subjectively chosen reference groups give direction to our lives.

Reference groups relate directly to achieved social status (such as professional groups) or to ascribed status (such as ethnic groups). Examinations of life-history data over long periods of time, or during specific transitions in social mobility, show changing sequences of subjective and objective affiliations with a variety of reference groups (Merton & Kitt, 1969).

## 8. Class

All micro and macro social structures and processes are anchored in social class, a series of groups which define membership according to specific criteria. Social class includes socioeconomic strata, classes of different age, gender, and other special interests (Dahrendorf, 1959). Classes are not formally organized and many people may not be aware of their class membership. In all instances, class exerts significant overt and covert influences on individuals' behavior. An examination of the power dimensions of different classes focuses individual efforts to see self in the context of social structures (Mills, 1956).

## 9. Culture

*Culture* is the conglomerate of social values within a particular society. Widely accepted values have more power in society than minority group or less-accepted marginal values. Individuals see their behavior differently when they analyze their transactions with others in relation to the dominant value patterns in society. We negotiate values and create culture; all our values are negotiated or not negotiated in the context of culture. Values define a population's quality of life and public issues, which are particularly significant during stressful periods and times of rapid social change. Ambiguities in values create burdensome complexities in the identity processes of individuals and groups.

## 10. Society

*Society* is used here as a metaphor to represent the broadest social structures, world views, or cosmologies with which an individual can identify. The degree of congruence between an individual's world view or cosmology, and the world as it actually exists in spiritual, mental, emotional, and physical dimensions, is a significant influence in determining the effectiveness of that person's behavior. Articulating a meaningful vision of the universe empowers self. Expanding awareness, through using a broad context to examine one's life, promotes the transcendence of empirical realities such as restrictive conditions. This broad conceptualization of society includes views of history and evolution, as well as the universe (Tielhard de Chardin, 1965).

## CLINICAL SOCIOLOGIST AS AGENT OF CHANGE

Applications of these concepts through clinical intervention and discussion increase clients' self-awareness and empower identity. Behavior is modified by changing perceptions of self and others and expanding definitions of reality. Patterns in interaction shift, and the client's relationships with broader social structures increase and become more flexible. One consequence of these modifications is that individuals become more autonomous, more able to choose or repeat specific roles. More predictable qualities of change in identity empowerment are listed here.

1   Clients become increasingly aware of their personal and social past and present.
2   They increase their options and choices in current everyday behavior.
3   They formulate more meaningful directions in their lives by examining their values in personal and social contexts.
4   Enhanced coping mechanisms and conflict resolution improve the quality of social relationships in the long run. In the short run, they may appear ineffective given intense resistance by those disadvantageously affected by the changes.
5   A clearer vision of society and the universe generates new goals and effective action for their attainment.
6   Attention shifts from personal troubles to social issues, and enlightened social action is realized (Mills, 1959).

## REFERENCES

Berger, P. L., & Luckmann, T. (1966). *The social construction of reality: A treatise in the sociology of knowledge.* New York: Doubleday.
Blumer, H. (1969). *Symbolic interaction: Perspective and method.* Englewood Cliffs, NJ: Prentice-Hall.
Caplow, T. (1968). *Two against one: Coalitions in triads.* Englewood Cliffs, NJ: Prentice-Hall.
Cooley, C. H. (1964). *Human nature and the social order.* New York: Schocken.
Dahrendorf, R. (1959). *Class and class conflict in industrial society.* Stanford, CA: Stanford University Press.
Garfinkel, H. (1967). *Studies in ethnomethodology.* Englewood Cliffs, NJ: Prentice-Hall.
Gerth, H., & Mills, C. W. (1953). *Character and social structure: The psychology of social institutions.* New York: Harcourt, Brace, and World.
Glassner, B. & Freedman, J. (1979). *Clinical sociology.* New York: Longman.

Goffman, E. (1959). *The presentation of self in everyday life.* New York: Doubleday.

Homans, G. (1961). *Social behavior: Its elementary forms.* New York: Harcourt, Brace, and World.

Lee, A. M. (1955). The clinical study of society. *American Sociological Review, 20,* 648–653.

Mead, G. H. (1934). *Mind, self and society.* Chicago: University of Chicago Press.

Merton, R. K., & Kitt, A. S. (1969). Reference groups. In L. A. Coser & B. Rosenberg (Eds.), *Sociological theory* (pp. 243–250). New York: Macmillan.

Mills, C. W. (1956). *The power elite.* London: Oxford University Press.

Mills, C. W. (1959). *The sociological imagination.* London: Oxford University Press.

Simmel, G. (1950). *The sociology* (Kurt H. Wolff, Ed./Trans.). New York: Free Press.

Straus, R. A. (1984). Changing the definition of the situation: Toward a theory of sociological intervention. *Clinical Sociological Review, 2,* 51–63.

Straus, R. A. (Ed.) (1979). Clinical sociology. *American Behavioral Scientist, 22* (4).

Swan, L. A. (1984). *The practice of clinical sociology and sociotherapy.* Cambridge, MA: Schenkman.

Teilhard de Chardin, P. (1965). *The phenomenon of man.* New York: Harper & Row.

Thomas, W. I., & Znaniecki, F. (1927). *The polish peasant in Europe and America.* (Vols. 1 & 2). New York: Knopf.

Thomas, W. I. (1931). The relation of research to the social process. In W. F. G. Swann et al. (Eds.), *Essays on research in the social sciences* (pp. 175–194). Washington, DC: Brookings Institution.

Wirth, L. (1931). Clinical sociology. *American Journal of Sociology, 37,* 49–66.

# Life-History Applications

*Ideal types* are theoretical models constructed from compilations of data from a wide range of complex life histories. They are used here to illustrate different kinds of identity, related behavior, and functioning. Ideal types represent patterns in the data, describing and defining different ranges and degrees of identity. Clinical and research data from several hundred detailed life histories are the sources for these identity typologies.

The primary source of life-history data and ideal type applications are special situations and experiences of women. It is assumed in describing outcomes that clinical sociological intervention strengthens clients' identity.

Ideal types may also be thought of as methodological tools for systematizing contrasts and similarities in identity processes, and as demonstrating a range of possibilities in identity and value choices. Although many more examples are possible, contrasts in strength of identity and within the context of denominational influence and spirituality have been chosen to portray the most basic cultural varieties found in Western society. Religion and spirituality are both viewed as sources of values for identity empowerment. Historically, women's lives have been markedly structured and restricted by family and religion, and these ideal types illustrate a cross section of possibilities.

Identity concerns are inextricably related to our interaction patterns and the meanings we assign values. The intensity and tenacity with which we cling to certain values influence our behavior as much as, if not more than, the meaning of the values we choose. Deep-seated values define our behavior and understanding of social trends. As our most sanctified values color our perceptions of reality, our value choices and related priorities are the foundations of our identity, commitments, and activities.

## STRONG IDENTITY

The strong identity ideal type illustrates effective self-empowerment through heightened awareness of value choices. Strong identity may be a given, or it may be achieved through self-strengthening activities undertaken independently or in a clinical context.

The major characteristics of the strong identity follow. Although these properties are manifested by both genders, they are discussed here in terms of their applicability to women.

1  Strong identity is clarity in value preferences and commitments.
2  Strong identity evolves from painstaking reflection and decision-making.
3  The core of strong identity is one or several values chosen to give direction and purpose to activity. Commitments are coordinated with the central values of strong identity.
4  Strong identity is characterized by the preeminence of activity over passivity, and by contribution or orientation to the common good.
5  Strong identity is flexible since the flow of life is experienced rather than predicted at every turn. Relationships and commitments are made sufficiently flexible to meet the needs of changing circumstances.
6  The direction and typical behavior patterns of strong identity are expansive rather than restrictive. Strong identity includes defining and pursuing opportunities for change.
7  Strong identity is awareness of values integrated with goal-directed behavior. Goals and commitments flow from values chosen as the core of identity.

## MODERATE IDENTITY

Moderate identity may be a given characteristic of self or a transition in self-concept resulting from clinical sociology applications. Some contrasting characteristics are noted.

**1**  Moderate identity frequently evolves from changing habits of reflection and behavior. Moderate identity is characterized by motivation to work towards clarity in value preferences and commitments.

**2**  Moderate identity is reflection and deliberation alternating with periods of automatic, nonreflective, and nondeliberate behavior. Decisions may be reactive and adaptive to others' demands and expectations rather than autonomous.

**3**  Moderate identity does not have a distinct core of values, but behavior generally shows fairly consistent value patterns. A person's values and behavior are fairly well integrated and coordinated through commitments, but moderate identity is not characterized by the same degree of decisive autonomy as strong identity.

**4**  Moderate identity is both active and passive, sometimes adapting to others' requests in self-destructive ways. Goals are vague in moderate identity, but they may be oriented towards contributing to the common good, especially under nonstressful conditions. Activity towards these goals enhances well-being and empowers identity.

**5**  Moderate identity tends to be overly rigid and unyielding in relation to others and changing circumstances. When this rigidity inhibits strengthening identity, growth will be stunted at moderate identity levels with no possibility of moving to strong identity.

**6**  Direction envisaged by moderate identity tends to be relatively narrow and restricted. Moderate identity is not associated with opportunist or pioneering patterns of behavior, but with relatively conservative postures that tend to endorse and support the status quo.

**7**  Moderate identity is less aware of values and goals than strong identity. Commitments may be contradictory in moderate identity, and these contradictions lead to ineffectiveness in interpersonal and social behavior.

## WEAK IDENTITY

Behavior that counteracts or detracts from identity formation results in weak identity. Weak identity is a particular combination of given characteristics or specific responses to crisis situations. Weak identity is frequently a starting point and presenting problem in clinical sociological therapy rather than a product of therapeutic intervention. As in the case of moderate identity, it is possible for weak identity to be reoriented towards strengthening identity, especially through support and direction in clinical intervention. Selected characteristics of weak identity are described here.

**1**  Weak identity is a product of automatic, reactive, and nonreflective behavior, devoid of a sense of self in interaction with others, and devoid of a sense of belonging to humankind. It results from emotional isolation. Weak identity is also characterized by adaptive, not self-motivated, behavior.

**2**  Weak identity is controlled by others and by others' values. It has no autonomy, but extends self for sacrifice, victimization, and other destructive processes. There is overcompromise and all values are negotiable.

3   Weak identity does not have a distinctive core of values. Values claimed vacillate, depending on circumstances and others' pressures. Effective commitments cannot be made as weak identity has no established priorities in values. Behavior is random, predictably dysfunctional, or destructive. Weak identity has little awareness of continuities or patterns and repetitions in behavior. Action is perceived as relating to a present which is separate from past or future.

4   Weak identity is essentially passive. Behavior that appears to be active is reactivity to pressures of the moment rather than planned, coordinated, or integrated activity. Weak identity cannot make and keep commitments effectively, except those that are so tradition-bound that they are prompted more by imitation than by conscious, deliberate decisions. Weak identity is devoid of goals or intention to contribute to the collective good.

5   Weak identity may be very rigid as well as open to the pressures and whims of others. Though some values are adhered to, especially those of traditional stereotypes, they are a restricting influence on everyday behavior. Rather than sustain strength, rigidly held values limit behavior. Only crises or deliberate choices to grow and change can break through this rigidity.

6   Weak identity has no interest or inclination to formulate direction or purpose in everyday activity. World views of weak identity tend to be static and restrictive, accepting the status quo rather than seeing other realities or possibilities in personal and social conditions. Weak identity does not entertain visions of optimal conditions, but rather focuses on problems in current conditions.

7   Weak identity is unaware of self, others, and sometimes of the world outside personal milieus. Weak identity becomes a pawn of the social system through overconformity or reaction to conflict. Societal conflicts are internalized as personal or interpersonal conflicts, and weak identity is vulnerable to scapegoating processes and subordination by others.


## PROTESTANT IDENTITY

Each religion defines a fairly coherent set of values, roles, and expectations for women, and a different set of values, roles, and expectations for men. Depending on the extent to which a religion is an established denomination rather than a sect, gender differentiated values, roles, and expectations reflect mainstream traditions in society. Religions have their own powerful sanctions and entrenched traditional values which have a conservative influence on the status quo.

Protestant identity for women reflects majority experience in the United States although secularization has eroded the salience of religion for many women. Protestant values have distinctive consequences for women and identity, and for the commitments women make. Some of these are listed here.

1  Protestant women worship patriarchal values through Christian traditions and practices that focus on individual conscience. Individuality and individual decision-making are endorsed by this belief system although expectations for women are generally restricted to family responsibilities and congregation participation.

2  Protestant values include hard work, but for women this industry is expected to be confined to the home and not expressed as direct contribution to society.

3  Protestantism values individual achievement as demonstration of the glory of God. Achievement for women, however, is thought of in domestic terms rather than economic or political terms.

4  Protestant emphases on conscience and individuality have increased women's sense of responsibility unduly, producing guilt and isolation from each other. Although women may not be active Protestants, or even nominal Protestants, these values are influential throughout the United States.

5  Protestantism is a predominant or mainstream religion in different Western societies. This influence legitimates the subordination of women on an international scale. Protestantism also reinforces secular values and social sanctions which restrict women's lives.

6  Protestantism exaggerates the importance of conscience in women's lives, and this value's effect on decision-making increases women's guilt about conflicts in social values that are not their own.

7  Although Protestantism is historically based on tenets which question and restate Roman Catholic doctrines and dogma, Protestantism now fosters unquestioning attitudes to authority. Protestantism provides answers to questions which are thought to be of ultimate concern, but Protstantism formulates these questions from its own frame of reference and basic assumptions. Women who question the institutionalized values of Protestantism and mainstream society are labeled as deviant.

## ROMAN CATHOLIC IDENTITY

Like Protestantism, Roman Catholicism is an established denomination. The highly complex international organization of Roman Catholicism is a more visible patriarchal value system than Protestantism. The garb and celibacy of Roman Catholic priests add to the distinctiveness of patriarchal leadership in Roman Catholicism.

Roman Catholic experience and identity for women result from overt male influences in the Roman Catholic hierarchy. Some of the ways in which Roman Catholic values define identity and commitments for women follow.

1  Roman Catholic women worship patriarchal values through long-standing Christian traditions which focus on unquestioning obedience to authority. Conformity to religious and secular traditions is endorsed through this belief system, and women are expected to be obedient to male authority in the family

as well as in the Church. As no major leadership roles are open to women within the Roman Catholic church, women must demonstrate their faith largely through devotional practices in the congregation and at home.

2   Roman Catholic values include the parenting of large families. Women are caught in parental expectations which are strongly endorsed by religious sanctions.

3   Roman Catholic beliefs are fostered through parochial education. Roman Catholic socialization of women is particularly deep, and subservience to men is valued more than freedom to search for objective knowledge or to acquire and express skills.

4   Roman Catholic prohibitions of birth control and abortion regulate central life concerns for women. Prohibition of remarriage after divorce adds further limitations and restrictions to women's personal lives.

5   Roman Catholic emphases on obedience limit women's development of autonomy. Women are not encouraged to strengthen or value their independent thought. Roman Catholic women are trained to follow male authority and male direction.

6   Roman Catholicism adds respectability to class position by honoring existing social structures. Roman Catholic values endorse the gender subordination of women.

7   The historical roots of Roman Catholicism are deep and the power of this religion is more clearly organized on a worldwide basis than Protestantism and Judaism. The pervasiveness and quantitative presence of Roman Catholicism gives Roman Catholic values more of a universal, omnipresent quality than Protestant and Jewish values. Women find it very difficult to challenge or modify the overwhelming influence of this patriarchal form in their lives.


## JEWISH IDENTITY

Judaism is the longest established denominational religion in Western society, but is generally a minority religion. Like Protestantism and Roman Catholicism, Judaism has a worldwide membership. Historically Jews have been persecuted more than Protestants or Roman Catholics. Due to these crisis conditions, the roots of Judaism are emotionally deeper than those of Protestantism and Roman Catholicism.

Jewish values endorse early patriarchal beliefs and practices. Traditional patriarchal families serve as models for contemporary relations, and many Jewish women are trapped in anachronistic religious and ethnic identities. Characteristics of these restrictions for Jewish women are described here briefly.

1   Jewish women worship anachronistic patriarchal values that are usually justified by history rather than in terms of personal meaning. Nonrational values are revered for their endurance rather than for meanings that transcend history. Women's lives are restrained by traditional, nonrational Jewish values.

2 Jewish values emphasize education. Education has freed many women, but traditional Jewish expectations for women tend to limit them to domestic arenas rather than encourage their participation in society. However, women can be rabbis or teachers within some groups of Judaism.

3 Jewish values focus on family life. Women's roles as wife and mother are sanctified by Judaism to a much greater extent than more active roles in society.

4 Jewish values perpetuate family bonds, and divorce rates are lower among Jews than Protestants. Although remarriage in Judaism is accepted more than remarriage in Roman Catholicism, informal sanctions against divorce keep women in unsatisfactory marriages.

5 Judaism encourages women to think independently and at the same time to be loyal to tradition. As a result, their freedom is conditional. Women internalize conflicts in expectations which inhibit their expansive living.

6 Judaism endorses women's social mobility through educational and occupational achievement. Paradoxically, women's status is expected to be disciplined by domestic loyalties. Women's family life is given a higher priority than their professional accomplishment. As personal achievement must follow commitment to family and religious traditions, Jewish professional women have a heavier burden of divided loyalty to career and family than women who do not have this deep emotional commitment.

7 The historical persecution of Jews has a strong impact on women's identity. Jewish women may not be comfortable with members of other religions or their secular peers. They tend to look to each other for models and support, and this may reinforce the ethnic sanctions which restrict their lives.

## SPIRITUAL IDENTITY

Spiritual identity transcends denominational religious identity and may synthesize different aspects of denominational identity. Spiritual identity incorporates values which relate to oneself, one's society, and the universe, these values being general rather than ethnocentric or parochial.

Spiritual identity places a high priority on truth, harmony, love, and life in daily activities and commitments. Some specific characteristics of spiritual identity, which contrast with the ideal types of identity described previously, are listed here.

1 Spiritual identity may be synonymous with strong identity in that central values espoused are clearly focused and acted upon in commitments. Moderate and weak identity can be strengthened and empowered by increasing spiritual awareness or transcendence in ordering personal values in identity. Spiritual awareness gives a broader view of one's life, and increases the possibility of objectivity in decision-making.

2 Spiritual identity synthesizes the most expansive and life-enhancing values of Protestantism, Roman Catholicism, and Judaism. It includes an aware-

ness of continuities in patterns of activity, as well as pioneering directions and attempts to cultivate new kinds of relationships and behavior.

3   Spiritual identity is tolerant and flexible, facilitating others' spiritual awareness and identity empowerment. It is spontaneous action within structures of meaningful commitments.

4   Spiritual identity promotes the transcendence of harsh empirical conditions. Women empower identity and move beyond restrictions and limits in their lives by developing a spirituality which supports and contributes to others.

5   Spiritual identity is characterized by an awareness of connections in the universe, and of visible and invisible realities. Identity is not isolated from others or from universal forces, and is part of a whole which is greater than personal, secular identity. It is an integral component of universal harmony. Conflictual negotiations of values with others may lead to qualitatively new patterns and harmonies, and different levels of spirituality.

6   Spiritual identity acknowledges a oneness with the human race and with life forces in the universe. It includes belonging with others without being limited or restricted by them, and it transcends reactivity by attributing meaning, purpose, and direction to relationships and activity.

7   Spiritual identity is experienced when all are believed to be equal participants in life. Women acknowledge their equal heritage and equal rights, allowing and supporting others in their equality. This equality promotes community and constructive contributions to society.

# Glossary

**Achieved roles**   Behavior and expectations related to a status gained through personal effort.

**Adaptation**   Conformity that makes survival possible, including internalizing values and beliefs that reflect external conditions.

**Alienation**   Structural conditions that result in overwhelming doubts about the ability to control one's life. Individual experiences of isolation, meaninglessness, normlessness, powerlessness, and self-estrangement.

**Anomie**   Social conditions under which expectations and rules of behavior are ambiguous or nonexistent. Anomie arises from value changes in society, such as transitions from traditional to modern institutions.

**Ascribed roles**   Behavior and expectations related to a status defined at birth. Individuals cannot control ascribed statuses such as race, sex, or age, and assigned expectations tend to be arbitrary.

**Androgynous values**   Values that both women and men honor. Androgynous values include syntheses of typically feminine and masculine values as well as gender-free values, such as knowledge, community activism, and autonomy.

**Assimilation**   The process by which subordinate or minority individuals and groups internalize the values and norms of the majority.

**Autonomy**     Freedom and independence of individuals and groups. The liberty to develop one's own values and to live according to one's own integrity.

**Awareness**     Conscious perception of oneself and one's situation. A deliberate effort to understand existing conditions and possibilities.

**Bonds**     Positive or negative attachments formed by frequent interaction and exchanges between two or more people.

**Bureaucracy**     Hierarchical organization with an extensive division of labor. Objective rules are applied through a stratified authority system.

**Cause**     A socially defined issue supported by a group of people who press for change in a particular direction.

**Choice**     Ability to select from available options; a necessary condition for fulfillment.

**Collectivity**     A group which has some degree of organization based on shared interests.

**Commitment**     Decision to orient one's life towards a particular goal or cause. Goals include relationships as well as activities.

**Community**     A group with some integrated values and concerns that transcend individual interests.

**Conformity**     Adherence to a particular set of norms established by a group or society.

**Connectedness**     Awareness of one's similarities with others, as well as an appreciation of each person's uniqueness; includes some responsibility for mutual well-being.

**Culture**     A group's shared beliefs, language, values, religions, and attitudes.

**Deviance**     Attitudes or behaviors that violate the cues and norms for behavior in a given situation.

**Dyad**     A two-person or two-group relationship characterized by patterns of subordination and superordination. An intrinsically precarious relationship since either party can withdraw temporarily or permanently.

**Dysfunction**     An inability to act effectively. Impaired or inappropriate response to others or particular situations.

**Egalitarian values**     Values based on the primacy of equality. Equity, equal worth, equal rights, and equal opportunity derive from the central value of equality.

**Empowerment**     A strengthening of individuals and groups through interaction on all levels of social organization. Empowerment begins with identity clarification and includes making commitments for action. Empowerment results from women assessing where they are and what they want to do.

**Enlightenment**     Quality of individual and group awareness that generates a new view of existing conditions. Enlightenment results from becoming more knowledgeable and acquiring wisdom.

**Equal opportunity**    Similar access to resources and the satisfactions of full living.

**Equal worth**    Attempts to systematize parallels in ways in which women's and men's work contribute to society. Assessments imply degrees of similarity in the value of unlike occupations.

**Equality**    A state in which women and men are treated fairly and similarly without regard to sex, race, or ethnic background.

**Ethnic group**    People who share language, religion, race, or national origin.

**Evolution**    Broadest view of social change based on natural history and the physical sciences. Time spans of gradual change are measured in geological units which are difficult to comprehend.

**Family**    An emotional unit of personal relationships based on kinship or contract. Several generations of family members influence one another's behavior. The nuclear family is the most intensely dependent group to which individuals belong.

**Friendship**    Reciprocal relationships where meaningful communications enhance awareness of self. Friends provide significant support for each other.

**Fulfillment**    Developed potential and high quality of life for each person. A necessary condition for cooperative community.

**Goals**    Objectives to which an individual or group aspires.

**History**    A documented account of the past, and an awareness of the past's influence on the present and future.

**Ideas**    Concepts which may be accepted or rejected.

**Ideals**    The intrinsic perfection of cherished values.

**Ideal types**    Abstractions from empirical data that characterize the main properties of phenomena. Ideal types do not exist in their own right, rather they are used to illustrate or assess trends and tendencies.

**Identity**    The essence of being, an affinity with one's most sacred values. Our deepest beliefs about human nature and the human condition are sources of identity. Identity is cultivated by individuals and groups.

**Identity empowerment**    Tool used by clinical sociologists whereby identity is experienced as volitional behavior. Identity is empowered by selecting preferred values as a basis for decisions and commitments.

**Interest**    A goal or purpose which reflects the most central needs and aspirations of an individual or group.

**Intransigence**    Refusal to compromise in negotiations with others.

**Isolation**    Lack of connectedness with others, a state of being that has no sense of belonging.

**Liberation**    Autonomy and freedom in behavior. Movement away from restricted milieus (such as families) to community and societal involvement and participation.

**Life-history data**     Facts in the social histories of individuals and families. Facts that span a whole lifetime and the lives of several generations.

**Longitudinal data**     Information gathered about the same individuals or groups over long periods of time. Data may represent critical stages or development phases during a time frame of 50 years or more.

**Meaninglessness**     Sense of being insignificant or unimportant. Lack of awareness of values so that one's life conditions seem absurd.

**Metamorphosis**     Radical transformation of one's values, commitments, and activities. Changing one's identity through increased awareness of values or new value choices brings about a dramatic shift in attitudes and behavior.

**Modern values**     Desired objectives that emerge during times of industrialization and technological change. Modern values include high material standards of living and professional accomplishments such as discoveries in science and medicine.

**Norm**     Behavior patterns defined and widely accepted by society. A shared cultural rule or guideline for individuals' or groups' behavior in specific situations.

**Objectivity**     Value-free observation and knowledge of the external world as experienced or measured through the sense.

**Opportunity**     Fortuitous conditions which can be used to acquire an advantage or favorable circumstance for action.

**Optimal conditions**     The most beneficial circumstances for particular activities.

**Paradigm**     A theoretical model with a particular set of assumptions, relationships, and outcomes. An abstract construct which implies correlations or explanations between selected variables.

**Parasitical functioning**     Extreme dependence between two people where one acts at the expense of the other. Symbiotic closeness in a relationship which impairs the free activity of each person. Physiological symptoms or behavior problems generally characterize this kind of activity.

**Patriarchal values**     The desired objectives of men embodied in traditional social institutions. Patriarchal values are based on male-dominated hierarchical authority systems which resist change. The substance of patriarchal values is masculine power and interests.

**Powerlessness**     Inability to articulate or achieve goals that one wants to achieve. Inability to control resources or other crucial aspects of one's environment.

**Priority**     Values or objectives which an individual or group holds to be most important. Deliberately chosen preferred courses of action.

**Privilege**     A combination of constructive life-chances where some have greater opportunities than others. Reliable access to political, economic, educational, or other resources.

**Productivity**     Ability to contribute to society and serve others effectively through community exchanges.

**Realization**    An awareness or understanding of one's life conditions that leads to productive activity and meaningful commitments. Self-knowledge translated into behavior that accomplishes valued goals.

**Reciprocity**    Mutuality expressed through shared values, negotiations, exchanges, and other kinds of interaction. Reciprocity is a basis of community life as well as family relations, where returns for contributions are expected.

**Reference group**    Significant others who express values or goals with which one identifies. A feeling of belonging to a reference group may influence behavior more than actual membership. Inner changes are correlated with shifts in reference group identification.

**Resocialization**    A process whereby individuals deliberately ignore values they do not want and cultivate preferred values. Resocialization is not an intrapsychic process, and changes in patterns of interaction are imperative. New values and beliefs are internalized in resocialization, or old values and beliefs are reordered.

**Responsibility**    Action which includes self-knowledge, the deliberate choice of options, and informed anticipation of consequences. Responsibility flows from autonomy in interaction, and expressly does not include blaming others for one's situation.

**Retreat**    Purposeful withdrawal from exchanges with others in order to reflect and see the broader picture of one's life course and situation. Retreat ideally leads to reentry and higher levels of community participation.

**Role**    Expected behavior linked to a particular status or cultural context. Membership in groups implies specific roles and obligations.


**Secularization**    Emergence of modern values through industrialization and technological change. Religious institutions become more peripheral in secularization, losing their dominant influence on people's beliefs, especially those who live or work in urban contexts.

**Self**    Concept and awareness of one's individuality in relation to others. Self is active and monitors value dimensions of perception as well as behavior. Self makes decisions about values, roles, and other concerns.

**Self-discovery**    Realization that one's self expresses particular values or qualities which one may or may not like. Self-discovery is possible only when a person has some self-knowledge.

**Social change**    Broad processes which bring about shifts in structural and qualitative characteristics of society. Social change occurs at different rates in different parts of society. Entrenched values are extremely resistant to change.

**Social class**    Groups which define membership according to specific criteria such as economic resources, age, sex, and ethnicity. Some social classes are more closed than others and mobility is less likely in closed social classes.

**Socialization**    The process whereby all individuals internalize some of society's values and cultural expectations. Socialization is not a deliberate internalization of values, although others may select specific values for transmission through the generations. Choices in perceptions are made to some extent, but dependencies strongly influence which values are internalized.

**Society**    The broadest social structure of a nation state. Society is a context for understanding history and values.

**Spirituality**    An awareness of the cosmos and self that transcends empirical reality.
Ability to recognize similarities in religions and science, and to orient self to infinity as well as purpose in everyday life.

**Standard**    Values used as principles or guides in behavior. A standard—such as
truth—has both local and universal characteristics and implications.

**Success**    Ability to live according to deliberately selected values and goals. Responsible action that contributes to society and results in personal fulfillment.

**Survival**    Continuity in adaptation, in spite of temporary or prolonged harsh circumstances.

**Symbiotic functioning**    Extreme and intense interdependence where one party is
eclipsed by the other. Although both are trapped in the close relationship, only one
may suffer from physiological symptoms or problem behavior.

**Symbol**    Cultural or natural object or specific activity that represents values or meaning. The empirical dimensions of a symbol are much less significant than the meanings attributed to it.


**Traditional values**    Values which have endured through time and which are directly
related to hierarchical authority structures in society. Traditional values are at the
core of basic institutions such as the family, religion, the economy, the polity, and
education.

**Transcendence**    Ability to maintain a vision of ideals and cherished values in spite of
everyday realities or harsh empirical conditions.

**Triad**    A three-person or three-group relationship which generally has two insider
and one outsider positions. A triad is the smallest stable social system and can be
independent or related to other groups.


**Uniqueness**    Distinctive qualities of individuals which make one person different
from another. Uniqueness is a source of genius, the full expression of difference.

**Universal**    A standard or characteristic which applies to all people at all times in all
places. A few universals apply to each race, sex, and ethnic group.


**Value**    An objective or goal which is desired or cherished. Values are shared by
groups, and an individual's values are necessarily extensions of group values.

# Index